Quick and Easy Cooking for Diabetes

Simple, healthy recipes for people with diabetes and their families

Azmina Govindji

Thorsons

An Imprint of HarperCollinsPublishers

Thorsons
An Imprint of HarperCollins*Publishers*
77–85 Fulham Palace Road
Hammersmith, London W6 8JB
1160 Battery Street,
San Francisco, California 94111–1213

Published by Thorsons 1997

1 3 5 7 9 10 8 6 4 2

© Azmina Govindji 1997

Azmina Govindji asserts the moral right to
be identified as the author of this work

A catalogue record for this book is available
from the British Library

ISBN 0 7225 3498 1

Printed and bound in Great Britain by
Caledonian International Book Manufacturing Ltd, Glasgow

Contents

Acknowledgements

This book has been published in collaboration with the British Diabetic Association. I would particularly like to thank their Head of Diet Information Services, Norma McGough, and the Home Economist, Louise Tyler. My appreciation also goes to Moya de Wet for her meticulous analysis of the nutritional content of the recipes. This cookbook was compiled at a time when I had my finger in too many pies(!), yet throughout this hectic time, my husband, Shamil, has supported the project with patience and a great deal of compromise. I would like to dedicate this book to him and my children, Bizhan and Shazia.

Introduction

People with diabetes need to eat healthily, but what should you do if you know very little about cooking? Are you fazed by cookbooks for people with diabetes that expect you to conjure up a healthy meal using lots of exotic ingredients, make a smooth white sauce and be a dab hand at pastry? With this book you will be able to have healthy meals by using culinary short cuts. Instant sauce mixes, bought pizza bases, frozen veggies and pre-cooked pastry are only a few of the tips which make these recipes so quick and easy. All ingredients are readily available from supermarkets, and most dishes can be on the table in under 45 minutes.

This book provides step-by-step guidance on healthy cooking for people with diabetes and their families. It incorporates the latest dietary guidelines from the British Diabetic Association. The recipes are especially designed so that they:

- include a variety of low-fat, high-fibre ingredients, as is recommended for people with diabetes
- contain starchy carbohydrate, which helps to keep your blood glucose (sugar) within a healthy range, and to fill you up
- give serving suggestions which will help you achieve balanced meals
- are quick and easy, requiring no special ingredients or elaborate and time-consuming cooking methods.

And what's more, there's no need for you to worry about adding up figures for carbohydrate, fat or anything else. You can choose a dish confident in the knowledge that it follows the principles of the diet for diabetes. Since diabetics need to eat a range of healthy foods, this book is ideal for all health-conscious people.

What is Diabetes?

When you have diabetes, the amount of glucose in your blood is too high because your body cannot use it properly. Glucose comes mainly from the digestion of starchy foods such as bread and potatoes, and sweet foods like confectionery and chocolate. A hormone called insulin helps glucose enter the cells where it is used as fuel by the body. If there is not enough insulin, or if the insulin you have is not working well, then glucose can build up in your blood. This causes the classic symptoms of diabetes: thirst and a dry mouth, passing large amounts of urine, loss of weight, tiredness, genital itching and blurring of vision.

There are two kinds of diabetes:

- *non insulin dependent diabetes* is the most common type. Here, the body can still make some insulin, but not enough for its needs. Non insulin dependent diabetes can be treated by diet alone, or by diet and tablets, or sometimes by diet and insulin injections;
- *insulin dependent diabetes* occurs when the body has a severe lack of its own insulin. It is treated by insulin injections and a healthy diet.

There is no cure for diabetes, and there is no such thing as mild diabetes. However, with the appropriate treatment, you can enjoy a full, healthy and active life.

The main aim of treatment is to avoid 'highs' and 'lows' in your blood glucose level. Together with a healthy lifestyle, this will help to improve your well-being and protect against long-term damage to your eyes, kidneys, nerves and heart.

Which Foods?

Diet is the most important part of your treatment. Whether you need to take medication or not, what you eat and how often you eat have a significant effect on your blood glucose (sugar). What you eat also affects the amount of fat (like cholesterol) in your blood. If you have diabetes, you already have an increased risk of developing heart disease, so watching what you eat is particularly important. Insulin or tablets are not a substitute for a healthy diet.

Making the Right Food Choices

- Eat regular meals based on starchy foods.
- Try to eat more high-fibre foods, particularly beans, peas, lentils, vegetables, fruit and oats.
- Cut down on fried and fatty foods such as butter, margarine, fatty meat and full-fat cheese.
- Reduce the amount of sugar you eat by swapping high-sugar foods for low-sugar alternatives.

- Try to get to the weight that is right for you and stay there.
- Be careful not to use too much salt. A high salt intake is linked with high blood pressure.
- Limit the amount of alcohol you drink.
- Avoid diabetic foods. They have no special benefit for people with diabetes.

There are lots of healthy-eating tips in this book. It's a good idea to pick out the changes that you feel will easily fit into your lifestyle, choosing foods you enjoy. And there's no need to think that there are foods you *must* eat and those you must not. Healthy eating is all about balance – choosing a variety of healthy foods you enjoy and not forcing yourself to eat foods you dislike.

Below are some suggestions for including healthier items in your diet. You may find that you already choose many of the recommended foods regularly, so eating well may be easier than you think.

STARCHY FOODS

Make starchy carbohydrate foods (such as bread, rice, pasta, cereals, chapatis and potatoes) the main part of every meal. This helps to promote slow, steady rises in blood glucose, which is desirable. You may like to serve extra bread with main meals to boost the carbohydrate. Many recipes in this book contain pasta, which is an excellent starchy food for people with diabetes. It is slowly absorbed by the body, so it will not raise your blood glucose levels too quickly. Starchy foods are also filling, and if they are cooked in the minimum of fat, they can be low in calories too.

Cutting down on meat and cheese portions at mealtimes and filling up on starchy foods instead can be helpful if you're trying to lose weight.

High-fibre foods include wholegrain varieties of bread and cereals and potato skins. Starchy, high-fibre foods such as bran-based cereals and wholemeal bread are especially useful in preventing constipation. A high-fibre diet is recommended for the whole family, but remember that it is important to drink more fluid when you increase your intake of fibre. Try to have at least six to eight cups of fluid (such as water or low-calorie drinks) each day.

Oat-based cereals such as porridge and muesli are high in soluble fibre. These foods are absorbed even more slowly than starchy foods in general, and they can play a significant part in keeping your blood glucose within a healthy range. They can also help lower your cholesterol. Try to use oats in recipes (such as Oatmeal Herrings, *see page 75*), or start the day with an oat-based cereal. Instant hot oats cereals do contain soluble fibre, but because the oats have been 'mashed up', they have less effect on slowing down the rise in blood glucose after meals.

It is important to spread your intake of starchy foods evenly throughout the day and to eat regular meals. This helps to reduce fluctuations in your blood glucose levels.

FRUIT AND VEGETABLES
These foods contain essential vitamins that are needed for health, whether you have diabetes or not. A diet that contains plenty of fruit and vegetables will provide more fibre, especially soluble fibre, more antioxidant vitamins and will usually be

lower in fat. The antioxidant vitamins – betacarotene (which is converted to vitamin A in the body), and vitamins E and C – have been linked to a lower incidence of heart disease, some cancers and gut problems.

People in the UK tend to eat less fruit and vegetables than the recommended daily amount of five portions (not counting potatoes). Try to choose at least three pieces of fruit and two helpings of salad or vegetables a day. Many of the recipes in this book include a large proportion of vegetables. Those that contain beans or lentils are particularly high in soluble fibre, which helps to control your blood glucose levels. Again, like the oats, try to eat these vegetables as whole as possible (as in Mexican Butter Beans with Rice, *see pages 88–9*) rather than puréed.

There's no need to buy fresh vegetables if you haven't got time to prepare them. Frozen varieties are just as nutritious. Try to cook them quickly in the minimum amount of boiling water. Better still, steam them and serve immediately to help preserve much of the vitamin content. To keep your fat intake down, avoid adding butter or margarine to cooked vegetables. If you need a dressing on salads, try a bought fat-free vinaigrette or simply use some lemon juice or low-fat natural yogurt. Flavour this with coarsely ground black pepper and fresh or dried herbs to your taste.

Drinking large amounts of fruit juice, even if it is unsweetened, may make your blood glucose rise sharply. This is because fruit juice is concentrated and the natural sugar in a liquid form is rapidly absorbed by the body. If you like fresh fruit juice, take it with a meal rather than on its own. Alternatively, dilute it or choose a sugar-free squash or diet drink.

FATS AND DAIRY FOODS

One of the key tips for eating well, whether you have diabetes or not, is to cut down on your fat intake. Saturated fat has been shown to increase the amount of cholesterol, a type of fat, in your blood. A high level of blood cholesterol makes you more prone to heart problems. Since people with diabetes are at an increased risk of getting heart disease, watching your fat intake is particularly important. Eat fewer foods that are high in saturated fat, such as full-fat milk and cheese, fatty meat, lard, dripping, sausages, pies and pastries.

Replace some of these foods with those high in mono- or polyunsaturated fat. For example, use small amounts of rapeseed, olive, corn or sunflower oil in cooking. Instead of butter or margarine, choose a reduced-fat spread based on these oils. There is now a wide variety of lower-fat foods available in supermarkets. Use reduced-fat versions of dairy products, such as semi-skimmed or skimmed milk, half-fat Cheddar cheese and low-fat yogurt. Note that reduced-fat products can only help you cut down on fat and calories if you don't eat more of them than the full-fat versions.

MEAT, FISH, NUTS, PULSES AND EGGS

These foods are rich in protein and many are good sources of vitamins and minerals, such as iron and zinc. Meat can be high in saturated fat, however, so it is best to choose lean cuts and to minimize the oil you use in cooking. Here are some tips on choosing healthy foods from this group.

- Select lean cuts of meat and trim off visible fat. Try to cook meat without adding fat by grilling, roasting and braising. Avoid using the juices from roast meat for gravy.
- Remove the skin from poultry.
- Grill meat products such as sausages and burgers and allow the fat to drain off.
- Eat fish twice a week and oily fish, such as salmon, herring and mackerel, once a week. Choose drained, canned tuna in brine rather than in oil – the former has half the calories!
- Nuts are an important source of protein if you are vegetarian. However, they are also high in fat and are best taken as an ingredient in a main meal (like nut roast) rather than as a snack, especially if you are overweight.
- Pulses such as beans, sweetcorn, peas and lentils are an excellent source of soluble fibre. Choose them regularly. They are cheap and nutritious and can make main meal dishes go further (as in Chilli con Carne, *see pages 44–5*).
- Eggs can be poached, boiled or scrambled instead of fried.
- If you rely on lots of convenience foods, look out for lower-fat versions of ready meals.

SUGAR AND SWEET FOODS

You do not have to give up sugar completely. Small amounts of sugar, when taken as part of a meal, do not have a detrimental effect on your blood glucose levels. Only drinks and foods that have sugar as the main ingredient need to be avoided, as they can make your blood glucose rise sharply, particularly if they are taken in between meals. The table below gives examples of how you can swap high-sugar foods for low-sugar versions.

HIGH-SUGAR FOODS	LOW-SUGAR OPTIONS
sugar	artificial sweeteners, such as aspartame or saccharin
squash and sugary soft drinks	sugar-free squash and diet or low-calorie drinks
sugar-rich puddings	sugar-free jelly; sugar-free, low-fat instant desserts; 'light' or lower-fat versions of tinned milk puddings and custard
baked goods	wholemeal scones and loaves, cakes made with reduced amounts of sugar – try using some dried fruit for sweetness
cream-filled and chocolate biscuits	plain biscuits such as oatcakes, Rich Tea or Marie
canned fruit in syrup	canned fruit in natural juice or water

ALCOHOL

If you have diabetes, there's no reason why you cannot enjoy a drink, unless of course you have been advised to avoid alcohol for another medical reason.

Observe the safe drinking limit for everyone: no more than 21 units a week for men, and no more than 14 units a week for women. One unit of alcohol equals half a pint of beer or lager, one pub measure of sherry, aperitif or liqueur, a standard glass of wine or a pub measure of spirits, such as vodka or gin. These are maximum recommended amounts – it's better to drink less. Try to space your drinking throughout the week and to have two or three alcohol-free days each week.

Alcohol can cause hypoglycaemia (low blood glucose) if you are taking insulin or certain tablets for your diabetes. Here are a few guidelines on alcohol:

- Avoid drinking on an empty stomach. Always have something to eat with a drink. If you have been out drinking, it is particularly important to eat something afterwards. This is because the hypoglycaemic effect of alcohol can last for several hours.
- Choose low-alcohol drinks in preference to those higher in alcohol. Avoid special diabetic beers or lagers as these are high in alcohol.
- If you enjoy spirits, try to use the sugar-free/slimline mixers.
- Drink less alcohol if you are trying to lose weight.

Watching Your Weight

If you are overweight, your diabetes will be difficult to control. Being overweight also makes you more prone to heart problems. If you need to lose weight, cut down on fat and sugar, as described above. The recipes in this book are lower in fat than traditional ones, and taking some tips from the ingredients and cooking methods will help you cut down on calories.

About the Recipes

The aim of these recipes is to show you how you can keep to a healthy diet without having to spend hours in the kitchen. The dishes have been created using convenient and healthier alternatives to standard ingredients, making them low in fat and sugar whilst being high in fibre. Meals are cooked in only a small amount of cooking oil and the oils chosen are unsaturated, for the reasons outlined.

Each recipe has been carefully considered for its nutritional quality. Every dish has been analysed for the amount of fat, saturated fat, calories and fibre it contains, to ensure that it is in line with the principles of healthy eating. There's no need for you to worry about adding up the figures from these calculations. Rest assured that the recipes are far lower in fat (particularly saturated fat) than traditional recipes, and that ingredients high in soluble fibre have been used wherever appropriate.

The serving suggestions are based on the nutritional value of each recipe, with ideas on how to boost the carbohydrate content of the meal. It also provides tips on vegetables to complement the dish. Although some dishes may already contain vegetables, it is a good idea to serve extra vegetables or salad.

Most recipes include a healthy eating note. This section gives quick information on the nutritional quality of some of the ingredients and how they fit into an overall healthy-eating plan.

When preparing meals, try to use only small amounts of salt. A high salt intake has been linked to high blood pressure. Choose good non-stick cookware so that you can cook in the minimum of oil without difficult washing-up!

British Diabetic Association

Living with diabetes is not easy! But with the right help and reassurance, there's no reason why you can't live life to the full.

The British Diabetic Association (BDA) has been helping people for over 60 years. We probably have the answers to most of your questions and have information on subjects such as hypos, blood glucose testing, holidays, travel, employment and insurance. All members receive *Balance*, the BDA magazine, every two months, keeping up-to-date with the latest developments.

The BDA runs children's holidays, family weekends and days around Britain, where you can meet other families and healthcare professionals. Talking to people who have been through a similar situation can often be very helpful. The BDA has over 450 local groups and branches throughout the UK which provide support and hold regular meetings and social events too. We have also opened regional offices in the UK to help improve the level of local support.

The BDA supports research to improve treatments and to find a prevention or cure for diabetes and its complications. Although dependent on voluntary donations, the Association is one of the largest single contributors to diabetes research in the UK.

The BDA represents you – campaigning for improved health care services and making representations to the Government on your behalf. Everyone is urged to join the BDA – the larger our membership, the greater our influence on your behalf.

Contact the BDA at 10 Queen Anne Street, London W1M 0BD. Telephone: 0171 323 1531. Registered Charity No. 215199.

Starters

This chapter contains quick and simple dishes to whet your appetite. Some of these first courses can also be served as light lunch or supper dishes, but should be accompanied by something starchy, such as a large chunk of crusty bread, so that there is enough carbohydrate in your meal. The recipes range from hearty Lentil and Carrot Soup to a lighter Smoked Mackerel Pâté, and you are sure to find many healthy choices that become firm favourites.

The starters are designed to complement the main courses. Those based on vegetables, such as Baked Tomato and Olive Salad, are a good source of fibre and vitamins A (betacarotene) and C. Try to have two large portions of vegetables every day.

Leek and Potato Soup

No peeling or chopping of potatoes, no puréeing, just an instant mash potato mix with a fresh leek and you're well on your way! The mix is similar to potato flour, and you can use it to thicken the soup to your desired consistency. The crunchy leeks contrast beautifully with the smooth potato.

Accompany this with some crusty bread, or transform it into a main meal soup by also adding cooked peas or beans and sprinkling some reduced-fat Cheddar on top.

Preparation and cooking time: 15 minutes
Serves 3
Freezing: suitable

1	tbsp oil
1	bay leaf
2	fresh leeks, thinly sliced
1	vegetable or chicken stock cube
pinch	tarragon
30g (1oz)	instant mashed potato
	salt and pepper

1) Heat the oil and add the bay leaf.
2) Stir in the leeks and sauté for a couple of minutes to soften them.
3) Make the stock cube up to 285ml (½ pint) with boiling water.
4) Add the stock and the tarragon to the leeks and bring back to the boil.
5) Remove the pan from the heat. Add the instant mashed potato and stir well to prevent any lumps from forming.
6) Season and serve.

Healthy Eating Notes

This is a time-saving recipe. Although mashed potato is more quickly absorbed than whole potatoes, you can add pulses to the meal to promote good blood glucose control. If you do have more time, use fresh potatoes cut into small chunks. Serve when the potatoes are cooked but not mushy. Whole vegetables (rather than puréed) will not raise your blood glucose level so quickly. See the main Introduction for more information on this.

Chilli Chicken Wings

I use ready-made crushed ginger and garlic from a jar for this recipe so that I spend less than 10 minutes on preparation. Just one bit of advice – serve with plenty of napkins!

Preparation and cooking time: 30 minutes
Serves 4
Freezing: suitable

12	skinless chicken wings
1 tsp	crushed ginger, from a jar
2 tsp	crushed garlic, from a jar
1 tsp	red chilli powder
1 tbsp	olive oil
2 tsp	honey
2 tsp	coarse-grain mustard
1 tsp	cider vinegar
	salt and pepper

1) Preheat the grill to medium. Line a large flameproof dish with foil.
2) Put the chicken wings into a bowl. Add all the other ingredients and mix well.
3) Arrange the wings in the dish, making sure they don't overlap.
4) Cook under the grill for about 20 minutes, turning once or twice during cooking. Serve hot or cold.

Healthy Eating Notes

Remove the skin from all poultry before cooking to reduce the fat content. When you need to use fat in cooking, choose oil high in unsaturated fat, such as olive, rapeseed or sunflower oils.

Cocktail Kebabs with Yogurt Dip

Each chunk of marinated chicken is threaded onto a cocktail stick and then dipped in a chilli-flavoured sauce. Although this is a starter, you can serve it as a main meal for two by stuffing the chicken kebabs into warmed (preferably wholemeal) pitta bread and smothering it with the dip and shredded lettuce. Yum!

Preparation time: 25 minutes
Cooking time: 10 minutes
Serves 4
Freezing: not recommended

200g (7oz)	skinless chicken breasts, cut roughly into 2cm (1in) cubes
	FOR THE MARINADE
2 tsp	olive oil
1 tsp	dried basil
1 clove	garlic, finely chopped or crushed
2 tbs	light soy sauce
	salt and pepper
	FOR THE DIP
2 x 150g (5fl oz) pots	low-fat natural yogurt
3	spring onions, green stems only, finely sliced
good pinch	red chilli powder

1) Mix the marinade ingredients together.
2) Put the chicken pieces into a bowl and stir in the marinade. Set aside while you prepare the dip.
3) Preheat the grill to high and line the grillpan with cooking foil. Mix the dip ingredients together and chill in the refrigerator.
4) Thread each chicken piece onto a cocktail stick and grill for about 10 minutes, turning once during cooking. Serve hot or cold with the yogurt dip.

Healthy Eating Notes
Low-fat natural yogurt makes an ideal base for a dip to accompany kebabs, chilli or curried dishes.

Lentil and Carrot Soup

Vegetable soups make ideal starters or light meals. A large chunk of crusty bread is the perfect accompaniment.

Preparation time: 15 minutes
Cooking time: 20 minutes
Serves 4
Freezing: suitable

1 tsp	corn oil
15g (½oz)	butter
1	onion, chopped
3	carrots, peeled and roughly chopped
140g (5oz)	red lentils
½ tsp	thyme or *herbes de Provence*
1 litre (2 pints)	vegetable stock
	salt and pepper

1) Heat a large pan with a lid. Add the oil and melt the butter in the oil over a low heat. Add the onion and sauté gently to soften.
2) Add the carrots and stir-fry for a few minutes.
3) Stir in the lentils, herbs and stock. Bring to the boil.
4) Cover and simmer for about 15–20 minutes, until the lentils are cooked. Season and serve.

Healthy Eating Notes
Carrots are a good source of betacarotene, which is converted by the body to vitamin A, an antioxidant vitamin.

Tuna Cocktail

This salad makes an ideal starter served with bread.

Preparation time: 15 minutes
Serves 4
Freezing: not recommended

1 tsp	tomato purée
1 tbs	reduced-calorie mayonnaise
1 heaped tbs	low-fat fromage frais
185g (6½oz) can	tuna chunks in brine, drained
½	green pepper, diced
1 tbs	chopped fresh dill
	black pepper
4 tbs	finely shredded lettuce
1	fresh lemon, sliced

1) Mix the purée, mayonnaise and fromage frais in a bowl.
2) Add the mixture to the tuna and green pepper. Season with the dill and pepper.
3) Divide the lettuce into four equal portions and place in the bottom of serving glasses.
4) Arrange the fish cocktail over the lettuce and chill. Just before serving, decorate with a slice of lemon.

Healthy Eating Notes
Use reduced-calorie mayonnaise instead of full-fat versions. Canned tuna in brine or water has half the calories of tuna in oil.

Smoked Mackerel Pâté

A delicious starter with wholemeal bread or toast.

Preparation time: 15 minutes
Serves 4
Freezing: not recommended

2	cooked smoked mackerel fillets (weighing about 100g or 4oz each)
140g (5oz)	low-fat fromage frais
2 tbs	chopped chives
1 tbs	lemon juice
pinch	cayenne pepper (optional)

1) Remove the skin from the fish. Break the skin into small pieces and mash with a fork. Be careful to remove any bones.
2) Mix together the fromage frais, chives, lemon juice and cayenne pepper (if used).
3) Blend the fish with this mixture using a fork. Serve chilled.

Healthy Eating Notes
The low-fat fromage frais makes a healthy alternative to cream cheese or double cream which is often used in pâtés.

Prawns with Apple and Cucumber

Preparation time: 10 minutes
Serves 4
Freezing: not recommended

40g (1½oz)	reduced-calorie mayonnaise
40g (1½oz)	low-fat fromage frais
200g (7oz)	frozen prawns, defrosted
1	apple, cubed
115g (4oz)	cucumber (around 7cm/3in stick), diced
1 tbs	raisins
pinch	cayenne pepper

1) Mix the mayonnaise and fromage frais together.
2) Add this dressing to all the other ingredients, except the cayenne pepper.
3) Divide the mixture into four individual serving dishes and sprinkle the cayenne pepper on top. Serve chilled, with bread rolls.

Healthy Eating Notes

Shellfish such as prawns contain cholesterol, but this is not harmful to your blood cholesterol. This is because blood cholesterol is more influenced by the amount of saturated fat you eat. Prawns are low in saturated fat.

Pork Satay with Peanut Sauce

Preparation and cooking time: 35 minutes
Serves 4
Freezing: not recommended

225g (8oz)	lean pork, cut into bite-sized pieces

FOR THE MARINADE

1 tbs	light soy sauce
1 tbs	Worcester sauce
¼ tsp	Chinese five-spice powder
1	clove garlic, crushed
2 tsp	sesame oil
1 tsp	honey
	salt and pepper

FOR THE SAUCE

1 tbs	crunchy peanut butter
1 tsp	lemon juice
2 tsp	desiccated coconut
¼ tsp	red chilli powder

1) Preheat the grill to a moderately high heat. Line the grillpan with foil.
2) Prepare the marinade by mixing all the ingredients together.
3) Put the pork into a bowl and coat with the marinade. Set aside.

4) Mix together all the ingredients for the sauce with 3 tbs of cold water.
5) Thread the pork onto wooden skewers and grill until cooked, turning frequently.
6) Serve hot or cold with the peanut sauce.

Healthy Eating Notes

Lean pork can be just as low in fat as any other lean meat or poultry. Keep the fat down by using only small amounts of oil when cooking, as in this recipe.

Garlic Bread

Ready-made garlic paste, French bread and a hot grill make this into a quick and easy aromatic starter which goes especially well with pizzas and pasta dishes.

Preparation and cooking time: 10 minutes
Serves 4
Freezing: suitable

20cm (8in) stick	of French bread
55g (2oz)	low-fat spread
1 tsp	garlic paste
¼ tsp	mixed herbs

1) Preheat the grill to medium.
2) Cut the bread into 8 diagonal slices. Toast on one side.
3) Mix the spread, garlic and herbs together.
4) Spread the garlic mixture evenly over the untoasted side of the bread.
5) Grill the flavoured side till lightly browned.

Healthy Eating Notes
It's a good idea to serve extra bread with meals to boost the carbohydrate. The trouble is that it's usual to add some sort of spread. This recipe uses low-fat spread, which helps to keep the fat down. Remember that garlic bread bought in supermarkets or restaurants is likely to be made with lashings of butter – not the best of starters if you're trying to eat healthily!

Stuffed Mushrooms

Preparation and cooking time: 20 minutes
Serves 4
Freezing: not recommended

8	large flat mushrooms (about 225g/8oz), stalks removed
30g (1oz)	Cheddar cheese, grated
1 tbs	chopped parsley
4	pitted olives, halved
	freshly milled black pepper

1) Preheat the grill to medium. Line the grillpan with foil.
2) Put the mushrooms into a frying pan. Add a little boiling water and cover with a lid. Cook the mushrooms for a couple of minutes only.
3) Drain the mushrooms and place them on the grillpan, rounded side down.
4) Mix the cheese with the parsley and use this to fill the mushrooms. Put half an olive in the centre of each mushroom and season to taste with the black pepper.
5) Grill for about a minute until the cheese has melted, and serve immediately.

Healthy Eating Notes
It's traditional to cook mushrooms in butter or oil, but you can simmer them in water without losing the flavour – and without the extra fat!

Florida Cocktail

Starters based on fruit and vegetables are much healthier than conventional starters such as pâtés and can help to balance a heavier main course. You can also serve this dish as a pudding – it contains fewer than 70 kilocalories a portion!

Preparation time: 10 minutes
Serves 4
Freezing: not recommended

200g (7oz)	canned pineapple in natural juice, drained, reserving juice
2	satsumas, peeled and segmented
115g (4oz)	seedless grapes, halved
2	kiwi fruits, peeled and sliced

1) Mix the prepared fruits together with 100ml (3fl oz) of the reserved pineapple juice.
2) Divide the mixture into four individual serving glasses. Chill and serve.

Healthy Eating Notes
Fresh fruit is an excellent source of vitamin C and fibre. Try to eat three pieces of fruit a day.

Baked Tomato and Olive Salad

A warming starter with a piquant flavour and lots of juices. Serve as a starter or light snack with plenty of French or ciabatta bread to mop up the juices.

Preparation time: 5 minutes
Cooking time: 10–15 minutes
Serves 2
Freezing: not recommended

2	large tomatoes, sliced (around 140g/5oz each)
10–12	pitted olives, halved
3	spring onions, sliced
½ tsp	dried oregano
	freshly milled black pepper
1 tsp	coarse-grain mustard

1) Preheat the oven to 375°F/190°C/gas mark 5. Lightly grease/oil an ovenproof dish.
2) Mix all the ingredients together and place in the dish. Cover with foil and cook until the tomatoes have softened (about 10–15 minutes).

Healthy Eating Notes
Red, yellow and orange vegetables, such as tomatoes, yellow peppers and carrots, are rich in betacarotene. This is converted by the body to the antioxidant, vitamin A.

Meat and Poultry Dishes

Everyone has different likes and dislikes when it comes to meat and poultry dishes. This chapter caters for all by including traditional British dishes interspersed with flavours from other parts of the world. Family favourites such as Cottage Pie and Beef Stew have been adapted so that they use healthier ingredients.

Most of these meals take a mere 20 minutes to prepare as they use shortcuts such as instant mashed potato and sauce mixes. Although more exotic dishes, such as Chicken with Cashew Nuts, are featured, there are no elaborate or time-consuming cooking methods. And you don't need to go to specialist shops for the ingredients.

It's a good idea to get into the habit of choosing lean meat and skinless poultry when shopping. Poultry in particular can make 'quick and easy' dishes. In some cases, you may find it more economical to buy poultry with the skin on – this can be easily removed during preparation. Cooking methods such as grilling and stir-frying in the minimum amount of oil can help you reduce your fat intake even further. Choose unsaturated oils such as rapeseed, olive, corn and sunflower. Using non-stick cookware means you need less oil to prevent food from burning or sticking to the bottom of the pan. It also reduces washing up!

You can make meat dishes healthier by adding beans and other pulses to recipes, as in Chilli con Carne. This makes the meal go further and increases the amount of soluble fibre, which slows down the rise in blood glucose (sugar) after meals. This helps to keep your blood glucose within a healthy range, which is one of the key aims in the treatment of diabetes.

Meat-based dishes served as a main course are generally low in starchy carbohydrate. Use the serving suggestions in this chapter to help you select appropriate accompaniments to create a balanced meal.

Ham and Broad Bean Salad

Accompany this light lunch or supper dish with a large chunk of crusty bread.

Preparation time: 10 minutes
Serves 3
Freezing: not recommended

115g (4oz)	cooked ham, chopped
420g (15oz) can	broad beans, drained
2	apples, cored and cut into bite-size cubes
large pinch	freshly milled black pepper
1 tbs	chopped chives
2 tbs	fat-free vinaigrette dressing
	a few lettuce leaves

1) Mix all the ingredients except the lettuce leaves together.
2) Line a shallow dish with the lettuce and spoon over the ham and bean mixture. Serve chilled.

Healthy Eating Notes
Choose fat-free salad dressings to add flavour without piling on the calories. Fat-free versions are readily available in supermarkets, or you can make your own using lemon juice or vinegar, a pinch of herbs and coarsely ground black pepper.

Chicken with Cashew Nuts

A familiar Chinese favourite cooked with traditional ingredients. To save time, I use a frozen pack of Chinese vegetables, which contains mangetout and baby sweetcorn. Choose whichever vegetables you prefer, fresh or frozen. To serve, some plain boiled rice or noodles is all you need.

Preparation and cooking time: 20 minutes
Serves 4
Freezing: not recommended

FOR THE CHICKEN

1 tbs	plain flour
	black pepper
2 tbs	light soy sauce
2	skinless chicken breasts (weighing about 350g/12oz in total), cut into bite-sized pieces
2 tsp	corn or groundnut oil
30g (1oz)	cashew nuts

FOR THE VEGETABLES

1 tsp	sesame oil
6	spring onions, cut into thick diagonal slices
1 clove	garlic, crushed
1cm (½in)	root ginger, chopped or crushed (optional)
455g (1lb)	frozen or fresh Chinese mixed vegetables
2 tbs	light soy sauce
½ tsp	Chinese five-spice powder or pinch black pepper

1) Season the flour with the pepper. Stir the soy sauce into the chicken and then coat the chicken in the seasoned flour.
2) Heat a wok or wide-based non-stick pan. Add the corn or groundnut oil. Stir-fry the chicken over a high heat until well browned (about 5–6 minutes).
3) Add the cashew nuts and continue to stir-fry for a couple of minutes. Remove the chicken and cashew nut mixture, set aside and keep warm.
4) Heat the sesame oil in the same pan or wok. Add the onions, garlic and ginger (if using) and stir-fry for a few minutes.
5) Add the vegetables, soy sauce and five-spice powder (or pepper). Stir-fry for about 5 minutes.
6) Return the chicken mixture to the pan and heat through for a few minutes to let the flavours mix well.

Healthy Eating Notes

Quick cooking, such as stir-frying, is an excellent way to preserve nutrients. Soy sauce contains a lot of salt, so there's no need to add more. Always serve stir-fried dishes with plenty of boiled rice or noodles so that you fill up on starchy carbohydrates.

Chicken Pulau

A one-pot Asian dish that is wonderfully spicy and aromatic. It contains chicken, rice and vegetables and is substantial enough for any appetite. For convenience, I usually use crushed ginger and garlic from a jar. If you prefer a less hot and spicy dish, remove the seeds from the green chillies during preparation.

All you need to serve with this to make a tasty low-fat meal is some fresh mixed salad and low-fat natural yogurt.

Preparation time: 20 minutes
Cooking time: 20 minutes
Serves 4
Freezing: not recommended

2 tbs	corn oil
1	onion, finely chopped
3 tsp	cumin seeds
1 tsp	crushed ginger
1 tsp	crushed garlic
2	green chillies, finely chopped
285g (10oz)	chicken breasts, skinless, chopped into bite-size pieces
140g (5oz)	low-fat natural yogurt
5 tbs	sieved tomatoes
285g (10oz)	frozen mixed vegetables
	salt
500ml (18fl oz)	boiling water
225g (8oz)	basmati or long-grain rice

1) Heat the oil in a large saucepan with a lid.
2) Add the onion, cumin seeds, ginger, garlic and chillies. Fry gently over a medium heat.
3) Increase the heat and add the chicken. Brown for about 5 minutes.
4) Stir in the yogurt, tomatoes, vegetables and salt. Simmer for a couple of minutes.
5) Add the boiling water and bring back to the boil.
6) Stir in the rice, cover and cook over a medium heat until the water is absorbed (about 20 minutes).

Healthy Eating Notes
The combination of rice, vegetables and lean meat in this recipe provides a good mix of starchy carbohydrate, fibre and vitamins whilst keeping an eye on the fat content.

Honeyed Drumsticks

Balance this dish by serving with some starchy carbohydrate, such as boiled new potatoes in their skins. Accompany these with a couple of servings of colourful vegetables, such as French beans and sweetcorn. Alternatively, this makes a great outdoor dish if served with some crusty bread and mixed salads.

Preparation time: 5 minutes
Cooking time: 45 minutes
Serves 2
Freezing: suitable

2	skinless chicken drumsticks
2 tsp	honey
2 tsp	sesame oil
1 tbs	soy sauce
1 tbs	Worcester sauce
	coarsely ground black pepper

1) Preheat the oven to 190°C/375°F/gas mark 5.
2) Line a small ovenproof dish with cooking foil and put the drumsticks into the dish.
3) Mix all the other ingredients together and coat the chicken.
4) Cook in the centre of the oven for about 45 minutes or until the chicken is cooked and the juices run clear when the chicken is pierced with a fork.

Healthy Eating Notes

Removing the skin from chicken significantly reduces the fat content. Using a small amount of honey, as in this recipe, will not be harmful to your blood glucose level.

Lemony Roast Chicken

Chicken portions on the bone are sealed in foil with fresh lemon slices, whole cloves of garlic and fresh basil leaves. Let the flavours develop in the oven while you prepare the accompaniments. To serve, add some Sesame Green Beans (*see page 107*) with a starchy carbohydrate such as Vegetable Rice (*see page 103*) or boiled new potatoes in their skins.

Preparation time: 5 minutes
Cooking time: 40–45 minutes
Serves 4
Freezing: suitable

4	skinless chicken portions on the bone (about 455g/1lb total weight)
4	cloves garlic, peeled only
15g (½oz)	packet fresh basil leaves
2	fresh lemons, sliced
	salt and pepper
2 tsp	olive or rapeseed oil

1) Preheat the oven to 375°F/190°C/gas mark 5. Cut pieces of foil large enough to wrap each chicken portion.
2) Place each chicken portion with one whole clove of garlic, a quarter of the basil, a few slices of lemon and seasoning onto a piece of foil.
3) Drizzle each 'parcel' with a little oil. Loosely wrap the chicken pieces and roast until cooked.

Healthy Eating Notes

Using fresh herbs and garlic to season dishes enables you to cut down on the amount of salt needed in cooking. Eating too much salt is associated with a greater risk of high blood pressure.

Chicken Liver and Fennel

Chicken livers have a delicate taste compared to other offal. Make sure you don't overcook the liver as it can then become tough. The fennel used in this recipe has a mild aniseed flavour. This recipe makes a good alternative to the standard 'liver and onions' dish. If you like sweet and sour flavours, pour in a few tablespoons of fresh orange juice just before serving. Try serving with Sesame Green Beans (*see page 107*) and boiled new potatoes in their skins.

Preparation and cooking time: 30 minutes
Serves 2
Freezing: not recommended

2 tsp	corn oil
225g (8oz)	fennel, halved and thinly sliced
	salt and pepper
1 tbs	plain flour
225g (8oz)	chicken livers
3 tbs	chopped parsley
1 tbs	red wine vinegar

1) Heat the oil over a moderately high heat. Stir-fry the fennel for about 3 minutes.
2) Add the salt and pepper to the flour. Use this seasoned flour to coat the liver.
3) Add the liver to the pan and cook very quickly for about 5–10 minutes, stirring gently from time to time.
4) Slowly mix in the parsley and remove from heat. Pour in the vinegar. This should make a sizzling sound – serve immediately.

Healthy Eating Notes

Liver is an excellent source of iron, protein and B vitamins including B_{12}. Drinking some unsweetened orange juice with it will help you to make more use of the iron in the liver. This is because the vitamin C from the juice helps your body to absorb the iron more efficiently. Serving this dish with vegetables and a starchy carbohydrate, such as potatoes, provides a balanced meal.

Pan-fried Turkey Breasts

Turkey is available all year round and is often cheaper outside the Christmas season. The turkey in this recipe has a wonderful charred appearance. You can serve with the traditional roast potatoes and Brussels sprouts, or use jacket or boiled potatoes and vegetables or salad of your choice.

Preparation and cooking time: 20 minutes
Serves 2
Freezing: not recommended

1 tbs	plain flour
½ tsp	paprika
½ tsp	Cajun seasoning
½ tsp	dried mixed herbs
	salt and pepper
2	skinless turkey breasts (weighing around 170g/6oz each)
2 tsp	corn or rapeseed oil

1) Mix the flour with the paprika, Cajun seasoning, herbs, salt and pepper. Use this mixture to coat both sides of each turkey breast.

2) Heat the oil in a non-stick frying pan. Fry the turkey over a medium heat on both sides for about 15 minutes until the turkey is fully cooked.

Healthy Eating Notes

Turkey breast, like other poultry, is very low in fat. Choose it in preference to fatty meats and make sure you remove the skin and cook it with the minimum of added fat.

Turkey Fricassee

The definition of a fricassee is a white stew of poultry and vegetables which are first fried in butter and then cooked in stock with the addition of cream and egg yolks. This recipe is adapted to keep the saturated fat down by using Greek yogurt and chicken stock to make an appetizing sauce for turkey, carrots and green peppers. Buy fresh turkey breasts from the supermarket or make this into a great Boxing Day treat using leftovers. Add a dash of white wine for that special occasion. Serve with boiled rice.

Preparation and cooking time: 40 minutes
Serves 4
Freezing: not recommended

1 tbs	plain flour
	salt and pepper
4	skinless turkey breasts (weighing around 170g/6oz each), cut into bite-size chunks
2 tsp	corn or rapeseed oil
1	onion, finely chopped
2	cloves garlic, crushed
1	chicken stock cube
3	carrots, diced
1	green pepper, diced
110g (4oz)	Greek yogurt
4 tbs	fresh parsley, chopped

1) Mix the flour with the seasoning and use this to coat the turkey pieces.
2) Heat the oil in a non-stick pan. Add the onion and garlic and fry for a few minutes to soften.
3) Make the chicken stock cube up to 250ml (9fl oz) with hot water.
4) Add the turkey to the pan and brown over a medium heat, adding a little of the stock if it sticks to the bottom.
5) Stir in the carrots and remaining stock. Cover and simmer for 5 minutes.
6) Add the peppers and allow to cook, covered, for a further 5 minutes.
7) Stir in the yogurt and parsley. Warm through and adjust the seasoning if necessary.

Healthy Eating Notes

Greek yogurt contains more fat than most other yogurts. However, it is substantially lower in fat than cream yet still has a rich, creamy flavour.

Beef Stew

Although the cooking time for this recipe is lengthy, it can be prepared in just 15 minutes then left to cook on its own. A large helping of mashed potatoes helps to mop up the flavoursome juices of this stew.

Preparation time: 15 minutes
Cooking time: 1 hour 15 minutes
Serves 4
Freezing: suitable

1 tbs	plain flour
	salt and pepper
455g (1lb)	lean beef, cut into 2cm (1in) cubes
1	onion, chopped
1	beef stock cube, made up to 550ml (1 pint) with boiling water
½ tsp	mixed herbs
310g (11oz)	frozen casserole vegetables

1) Season the flour with the salt and pepper.
2) Coat the beef with the seasoned flour.
3) Brown the meat over a medium heat in a flameproof casserole dish.
4) Add the onion, stock and herbs. Cover and simmer till the meat is almost cooked (about an hour).
5) Stir in the frozen vegetables. Cover and cook for a further 10 minutes.

Healthy Eating Notes

It's perfectly acceptable to eat meat if you have diabetes, but try to choose lean meat to help keep the fat content down.

Beef Curry

When you think about preparing a curry, you imagine that you'll be slaving over a hot stove for hours. This quick and easy method needs only one pan and a bit of stirring. Otherwise, just leave it to cook on its own while the flavours develop and the aroma just manages to escape from a tightly closed lid. Complement this dish with some plain boiled rice, a large portion of mixed salad and some Cucumber and Mint Raita (*see page 124*).

Preparation time: 10 minutes
Cooking time: 20 minutes
Serves 4
Freezing: suitable

1 tbs	corn oil
1 tsp	crushed ginger, from a jar
1 tsp	crushed garlic, from a jar
2	fresh green chillies, chopped
1 tsp	turmeric
1 heaped tsp	curry powder
455g (1lb)	rump steak, cut into bite-size pieces
115g (4oz)	canned chopped tomatoes
2 tsp	tomato purée
125ml (4fl oz)	hot water
	salt
15g (½oz)	packet fresh coriander, chopped

1) Heat a large non-stick saucepan with a lid. Add all the ingredients except the coriander one at a time, stirring after every few additions.
2) Cover and cook over a medium heat for about 20 minutes, stirring occasionally until the steak is tender.
3) Stir in the coriander, heat through and serve.

Healthy Eating Notes
Choose lean beef wherever possible. This will help you to limit the amount of saturated fat you eat. If you want to make this dish go further, add 340g (12oz) of peas 10 minutes before the end of the cooking time.

Spicy Lamb Burgers

These burgers are tastier than shop-bought varieties, with much less fat. Serve with a large helping of salad and a large bap or if you're feeling really hungry some Southern Fries (*see page 112*).

Preparation time: 15 minutes
Cooking time: 15–20 minutes
Serves 4
Freezing: not recommended

FOR THE BURGERS

340g (12oz)	lean minced lamb
1	onion, grated
1	egg, beaten
2 slices	fresh wholemeal made into breadcrumbs
2 tsp	curry powder
¼ tsp	red chilli powder, or as desired
¼ tsp	mustard
	pinch of salt

FOR SERVING

4	burger buns, warmed
4	crisp lettuce leaves, washed and dried on kitchen paper
3	tomatoes, sliced

1) Preheat the grill to medium. Mix together all the burger ingredients.
2) Divide the mixture into 4 portions and form into burger rounds a little larger than the buns.
3) Place directly onto the rack of the grillpan. Grill for about 15–20 minutes or until cooked thoroughly, turning the burgers halfway through cooking time.
4) Serve in warmed buns filled with the lettuce and tomatoes.

Healthy Eating Notes

Choose lean minced lamb to keep your fat intake down. Grilling helps to drain off excess fat from the burgers as they cook.

Cottage Pie

This real family favourite can be time-consuming to prepare, but here's a way of speeding things up. Serve with a large portion of steamed or boiled vegetables or try it with Peas with Shallots (*see page 111*).

Preparation time: 20 minutes
Cooking time: 35 minutes
Serves 4
Freezing: not recommended

395g (14oz)	lean minced beef
1	onion, finely chopped
1	beef stock cube, made up to 200ml (7fl oz) with boiling water
1 tbs	Worcester sauce
200g (7oz)	canned chopped tomatoes in tomato juice
3	carrots, peeled and diced
	salt and pepper
126g (4½oz) packet	instant mashed potato mix
30g (1oz)	low-fat spread

1) Preheat the oven to 190°C/375°F/gas mark 5. Lightly grease an ovenproof dish.
2) Brown the mince with the onions in a large non-stick pan with a lid.
3) Add the stock, Worcester sauce, tomatoes, carrots and seasoning. Cover and simmer for 15 minutes.
4) Meanwhile, make up the mashed potato with boiling water according to instructions on the packet. Stir in the low-fat spread and season.
5) Put the meat mixture into the ovenproof dish. Spoon the potato mixture on top. Ripple the top of the potato with a fork and bake near the top of the oven for around 30 minutes until cooked.

Healthy Eating Notes

Cottage pie is traditionally quite high in fat. When you use a non-stick pan to cook the beef, there's no need to add extra oil. If you want to cut down even further, strain the excess fat from the mince after browning.

Chilli con Carne

This traditional Mexican meal of beef and beans is an ideal winter warmer. It has a hot, spicy flavour, which comes from the red chilli powder. Adjust this to suit your personal taste. I like to add some fresh coriander towards the end of cooking to give colour and a wonderful flavour. Serve straight from the dish with plenty of boiled rice, crusty bread and fresh green salad.

Preparation time: 20 minutes
Cooking time: 40 minutes
Serves 4
Freezing: suitable

455g (1lb)	lean minced beef
1	onion, chopped
1	clove garlic, crushed
2 tbs (30ml/1fl oz)	tomato purée
400g (14oz)	canned chopped tomatoes in tomato juice
1–2 tsp	red chilli powder
	salt and freshly milled black pepper
425g (15oz) can	red kidney beans, drained
15g (½oz) packet	fresh coriander, chopped

1) Brown the mince with the onion and garlic in a non-stick pan.
2) Stir in the tomato purée, tomatoes, chilli powder and seasoning. Bring to the boil.
3) Cover the pan and cook over a medium heat for about 30 minutes. Add a little hot water halfway through cooking if the mince begins to stick to the bottom of the pan.
4) Stir in the kidney beans and cook for a further 5–10 minutes. Add the coriander, adjust the seasoning and serve.

Healthy Eating Notes
Adding pulses like kidney beans to meat dishes is an excellent way to help the dish go further. It also increases the soluble fibre, which helps to improve your blood glucose levels and to lower blood cholesterol, a type of fat.

Pork with Spiced Apple

The tartness of cooking apples blends well with pork in this dish.
Delicious served with mashed or jacket potatoes and green vegetables or salad.

Preparation time: 20 minutes
Cooking time: 25–30 minutes
Serves 4
Freezing: suitable

2 tbs	plain flour
	salt and pepper
565g (1¼lb)	lean pork fillet, cut into cubes
2 tsp	corn oil
140ml (¼ pint)	dry white wine (optional) or juice of a lemon
2 tsp	ground cumin
½ tsp	mixed spice
1	chicken stock cube, made up to 200ml (7fl oz) with boiling water
2	cooking apples, cored and sliced

1) Season the flour with the salt and pepper and use it to coat the pork.
2) Heat the oil in a non-stick pan with a lid. Sauté the pork in the pan for about 5 minutes.
3) Stir in the wine or lemon juice, cumin, mixed spice and chicken stock. Bring to the boil. Cover and simmer for about 15 minutes.
4) Add the apple. Cover and cook for a further 10–15 minutes until the pork is fully cooked.

Healthy Eating Notes

Choose lean pork fillets or steaks. Lean pork is just as low in fat as other lean meats. To keep your fat intake down, try to use the minimum of oil in cooking.

Sweet and Sour Pork

Serve with plenty of boiled rice or noodles.

Preparation and cooking time: 20 minutes
Serves 4
Freezing: suitable

350g (12oz)	lean pork tenderloin fillet, cut into
	1cm (½in) cubes
1 tbs	cornflour
1 tbs	corn oil
1 tbs	light soy sauce
1	green pepper, cut into strips

FOR THE SAUCE

1 tbs	cornflour
2 tsp	caster sugar
1 tbs	white wine vinegar
2 tbs	fresh orange juice
1 tbs	light soy sauce
2 tsp	tomato purée

1) Coat the pork in the cornflour. Heat the oil in a non-stick pan. Fry the pork cubes over a high heat for about 5 minutes until brown. Add a little hot water if they begin to burn.
2) Stir in the soy sauce and green peppers and cook for a few minutes
3) Mix the sauce ingredients together with 3 tbsp of water. Add the sauce to the pan and stir until it thickens. Add a little hot water if you prefer the sauce to be less thick.

Healthy Eating Notes
Sweet and sour dishes can be high in fat and sugar. This is because the pork is often fried in batter and a lot of sugar is used in the sauce. In this recipe, instead of batter, the pork is stir-fried in a little oil and its own juices.

Tagliatelle with Ham and Cream

A rich-tasting Italian dish made with fresh basil and garlic. Serve with a large salad in fat-free dressing, and try not to have a high-fat starter.

Preparation and cooking time: 20 minutes
Serves 3
Freezing: suitable

200g (8oz)	tagliatelle
2 tsp	oil
1	onion, finely sliced
2	cloves garlic, crushed
200g (8oz)	mushrooms, sliced
90ml (3fl oz)	half-fat single cream
115g (4oz)	cooked ham, chopped
15g (½oz) packet	fresh basil leaves, chopped
	salt and pepper

1) Cook the pasta according to the instructions on the packet.
2) Heat the oil in a large non-stick pan over a medium heat. Add the onion and garlic and cook for a couple of minutes to soften.
3) Add the mushrooms and stir-fry for a few minutes until just cooked.
4) Pour in the cream. Add the drained pasta, ham, basil and seasoning and stir well. Heat through and serve.

Healthy Eating Notes

Pasta dishes are filling and nutritious, and although this is a rich dish, it uses half-fat cream as opposed to standard full-fat versions.

Fish Dishes

Fish is today's convenience food – it is versatile, cooks quickly, comes in a variety of shapes and sizes and can be served in many different ways. As you'll see from the recipes in this chapter, fish blends well with a range of different flavours. Choose herbs such as parsley and dill, as in Cod in Parsley Sauce, or if you prefer a bit more spice, try Tandoori Prawns.

Countries where fish is eaten widely have low rates of heart disease. Scientific studies suggest that oily fish eaten regularly may give some protection against heart problems. The special 'omega–3' oils which come from fish have been shown to lower blood fats such as cholesterol. It is thought that omega–3 oils also help blood to flow more easily round the body by making it less sticky.

Oil-rich fish, such as mackerel and herring, are high in omega–3 oils. This type of fish is naturally moist and needs no added oil for basting or cooking; just use a little lemon juice. White fish, such as cod and plaice, are low in fat. However, all types of fish are a valuable source of protein and are low in saturated fat. Try to eat fish twice a week, with one of these choices being an oily fish.

Cod in Parsley Sauce

Worried about lumpy sauces – or sticky washing up? This cheats' parsley sauce requires no cooking and yet has a wonderful creamy texture. Serve with boiled rice and salad, or new potatoes in their skins and vegetables.

Preparation time: 10 minutes
Cooking time: 20 minutes
Serves 4
Freezing: suitable

1 tbs	plain flour
	salt and pepper
4	cod fillets (weighing around 170g/6oz each)
1	onion, finely chopped
295g (10½oz) can	half-fat condensed mushroom soup
3 tbs	lemon juice
4 tbs	fresh parsley, chopped
4	tomatoes, sliced

1) Preheat the oven to 190°C/375°F/gas mark 5. Mix the flour with the seasoning and use this to coat each fillet.
2) Arrange the fish in a single layer at the bottom of a greased ovenproof dish.
3) Cover the fish with a layer of onion.
4) Mix the soup with the lemon juice and parsley. Pour this sauce over the fish and top with sliced tomatoes. Bake in the centre of the oven for 20 minutes till the fish is cooked.

Healthy Eating Notes

Choose fish in preference to fatty meats, and try to eat it twice a week. White fish such as cod is low in fat and ideal if you want to keep the calories down.

Mediterranean Fish

The aroma of bay leaves, garlic and basil … the bright colours of peppers and tomatoes … the flavours of lightly cooked fish, olive oil and herbs – a true taste of the Mediterranean. The delicious juices in this dish are best 'mopped up' with lots of French bread, mashed potato or boiled brown rice. Add a side salad to complete the meal.

Preparation time: 10 minutes
Cooking time: 30–40 minutes
Serves 2
Freezing: suitable

2	haddock fillets (weighing around 150g/6oz each)
½	green pepper, sliced
3	tomatoes, sliced
1	small onion, finely chopped
1	clove garlic, crushed
1 tbsp	olive oil
2 tbs	balsamic vinegar or lemon juice
1	bay leaf
1 heaped tbs	chopped parsley
½ tsp	dried basil
	salt and pepper

1) Preheat the oven to 375°F/190°C/gas mark 5. Lightly grease a shallow ovenproof dish.
2) Place the fish in the dish and add all the other ingredients. Stir gently and cover the dish with foil.
3) Bake in the centre of the oven until the fish is cooked.

Healthy Eating Notes

The traditional ingredients of the Mediterranean diet – fish, olive oil, garlic, lots of fruit and vegetables, red wine – have been associated with a reduced rate of heart disease.

Fish Pie

A warming meal which is made quick and easy by using an instant sauce mix. No need to cook the fish before baking in the oven. All the ingredients are simply mixed together and left to cook. Serve with some crusty bread and extra vegetables. Broccoli or spinach go particularly well with fish.

Preparation time: 20 minutes
Cooking time: 35–40 minutes
Serves 4
Freezing: not recommended

680g (1½lb)	potatoes, scrubbed and thinly sliced
4	frozen fish fillets e.g. haddock or cod (around 455g/1lb in total weight)
225g (8oz)	frozen peas
	salt and pepper
20g (¾oz) packet	parsley sauce mix
275ml (½ pint)	skimmed milk
50g (2oz)	reduced-fat Cheddar cheese

1) Preheat the oven to 220°C/425°F/gas mark 7. Lightly grease a shallow ovenproof dish, large enough for the fish to be placed in one layer.
2) Cook the potatoes in lightly salted boiling water for 5 minutes. Drain.
3) Place the fish and peas into the dish. Season lightly.
4) Make up the sauce, using skimmed milk, according to the instructions on the packet.
5) Pour the sauce over the fish and peas.
6) Layer the potato slices over the sauce.
7) Sprinkle the cheese over the potatoes. Bake in the centre of the oven for 30–35 minutes.

Healthy Eating Notes

Choose a mix which needs added milk, not water. This way, you can use skimmed milk to help keep the fat content down. Those mixes which require water often contain added fat.

Blackened Fish

Food from the Deep South of the United States has this classic blackened appearance. Blackened fish and chicken are becoming increasingly popular on restaurant menus in the UK. This recipe uses Cajun seasoning which is a unique blend of chillies, pepper, ginger and other spices. It comes ready mixed in a jar and you'll find it at the dried herbs counter in supermarkets.

The recipe needs virtually no preparation. Simply keep an eye on the pan and turn the fish a couple of times during cooking. Note that most bought frozen fish is usually best cooked from frozen. Check the label to see if defrosting is recommended.

Blackened fish goes well with boiled or baked potatoes or plain boiled rice. Remember to serve it with some vegetables – broccoli or French beans give a good contrasting colour.

Preparation and cooking time: 20 minutes
Serves 2
Freezing: not recommended

1 tbsp	oil
1–2 tsp	Cajun spice, as desired
2	frozen haddock portions or fillets (weighing around 100g/4oz each)

1) Heat the oil in a non-stick frying pan.
2) Sprinkle the Cajun spice liberally over one side of each piece of fish. Place the fish, seasoned side down, into the hot oil.
3) Sprinkle the top of the fish with the remaining Cajun spice. Turn the fish over after about 5 minutes. Cook the other side and turn again just to make sure the fish is cooked through. Serve immediately.

Healthy Eating Notes

Although it is best to cut down on fat and oil in cooking, you can pan-fry using very little oil. Choose oil high in unsaturated fat, such as olive, rapeseed or sunflower oils. Pat the fish with kitchen towel to remove excess oil.

Jumbo Salmon Fish Cakes

Serve these hot with baked beans or with a salad and home-made Salsa Sauce (*see page 123*).

Preparation time: 25 minutes
Cooking time: 10 minutes
Makes 6
Freezing: not recommended

126g (4½oz) packet	instant mashed potato mix
225g (8oz)	canned red salmon
2 tbs	chopped fresh dill
1 tbs	lemon juice
	salt and pepper
1 tbs	corn oil, plus a little for greasing
1	egg, beaten
115g (4oz)	cornflakes, crushed

1) Preheat the grill to high.
2) Make up the mashed potato according to the instructions on the packet. Mix in the salmon, dill, lemon juice and seasoning.
3) Divide the mixture into six portions and form each portion into a fish cake.
4) Line the grillpan with foil and brush some oil over the foil.
5) Dip each fish cake into the beaten egg and then into the crushed cornflakes.
6) Arrange the coated fish cakes on the greased foil.
7) Drizzle the remaining tablespoon of oil over the fish cakes. Grill for 10 minutes, turning once halfway through cooking.

Healthy Eating Notes

Fish cakes are usually fried. Even shallow frying will make the fish cakes absorb far more fat than that used in this recipe. For a higher-fibre recipe, you can use wholemeal breadcrumbs or branflakes instead of the cornflakes.

Salmon in Cream and Mustard Sauce

A special dish for entertaining and dinner parties made from lightly poached salmon and half-fat crème fraîche. Serve with boiled new potatoes and vegetables. Delicious with whole French beans and carrots.

Preparation and cooking time: 20 minutes
Serves 4
Freezing: not recommended

600g (1½lb)	salmon fillet, cut into 4 portions
	a few sprigs fresh parsley
1	bay leaf
3 tbs	lemon juice
6	peppercorns
	FOR THE SAUCE
170g (6oz)	half-fat crème fraîche
1 tsp	coarse grain mustard
2 tbs	fresh chopped dill or 1 tsp dried dill weed
	salt and coarsely ground black pepper
1	fresh lemon, quartered

1) Place the fish, parsley, bay leaf, lemon juice and peppercorns in lightly salted boiling water. Bring to the boil and simmer for about 10–12 minutes or until the fish flakes when tested with a fork.
2) Lift out the cooked fish with a perforated spoon.
3) Strain the liquid and add 4 tbs to the crème fraîche. Put into a frying pan and heat gently till boiling. Add the mustard, dill and seasoning. Heat through and pour the sauce over the fish. Serve with fresh lemon.

Healthy Eating Notes

Dairy products are everyday foods, so choosing lower-fat versions can help you cut down on fat. Examples are reduced-fat spread, reduced-fat cheese, skimmed and semi-skimmed milk and low-fat yogurt.

Tuna and Sweetcorn Pie

A single-crust pie which uses ready-made shortcrust pastry and a filling that needs no prior cooking. I often have the ingredients to hand for times when those unexpected guests arrive – and it only takes 20 minutes to prepare. Serve cold with a mixed salad and French bread or, as I prefer it, hot with lightly cooked vegetables and new potatoes in their skins.

Preparation time: 20 minutes
Cooking time: 20–30 minutes
Serves 6
Freezing: suitable

170g (6oz)	wholemeal shortcrust pastry, thawed if frozen

FOR THE FILLING

200g (7oz)	medium-fat soft cheese
60ml (2fl oz)	skimmed milk
200g (7oz) can	tuna in brine or water, drained
200g (7oz)	frozen sweetcorn
200g (7oz)	canned red kidney beans, drained
½ tsp	dried dill weed
½ tsp	dried basil
	salt and pepper

1) Preheat the oven to 375°F/190°C/gas mark 5. Lightly grease an ovenproof pie-dish. Roll out the pastry onto a floured surface so that it is large enough to cover the top of the dish.

2) Mix together the filling ingredients and put into the greased dish. Brush the rim of the dish with water (this helps the pastry to stay in place). Lay the pastry over the rim, taking care not to stretch it. Make a hole in the middle for the steam to escape.

3) Bake in the centre of the oven for 20–30 minutes or until the pastry is golden.

Healthy Eating Notes

Drained tuna in brine or water has around half the calories of drained tuna in oil. If you want to get the fat even lower, try using skimmed milk soft cheese (quark) instead of the medium-fat cheese.

Prawn Pilaff

A pilaff is an Eastern method of cooking rice with various spices. You can serve it alongside a main dish, as you would do with potatoes. Alternatively, it can be served as a main course if it is made with fish or chicken, as in this recipe. Although the list of spices in the ingredients may seem elaborate, you'll find they are very versatile and can be used to flavour leftovers. And this pilaff, surprisingly, takes only 15 minutes to prepare. Serve with some low-fat natural yogurt (such as Raita, *see page 124*) and Tomato and Coriander Salad (*see page 121*).

Preparation time: 15 minutes
Cooking time: 20 minutes
Serves 4
Freezing: not recommended

225g (8oz)	long-grain rice
1 tbsp	corn oil
2 tsp	cumin seeds
2 tsp	coriander seeds
1	onion, sliced lengthways
2 tsp	crushed garlic (from a jar or tube)
2	tomatoes, chopped
½ tsp	turmeric
¼ tsp	salt
170g (6oz)	fresh or frozen prawns, defrosted if necessary
200g (7oz)	frozen peas
500ml (18fl oz)	boiling water

1) Rinse the rice and soak in plenty of cold water.
2) Heat the oil in a large non-stick pan with a lid. Add the cumin, coriander, onion and garlic, and stir-fry for a few minutes to soften.
3) Add the tomatoes, turmeric and salt. Cook till the tomatoes are mushy, stirring occasionally.
4) Add the prawns and peas with the boiling water. Bring back to the boil, lower the heat, cover and simmer till the rice is cooked (about 15–20 minutes). All the water should be absorbed.

Healthy Eating Notes
Prawns are much lower in fat than meat and poultry.

Prawn Chow Mein

A quick and easy stir-fry recipe which looks impressive at a dinner party or is easy enough to prepare any day of the week. The noodles in this dish provide starchy carbohydrate.

Preparation and cooking time: 20 minutes
Serves 4
Freezing: not recommended

2 tsp	corn oil
1	large onion, sliced lengthways
1cm (½ inch)	root ginger, chopped or crushed
200g (7oz)	fresh or frozen prawns, defrosted if necessary
¼ tsp	Chinese five-spice powder
115g (4oz)	beansprouts
340g (11oz)	frozen sweetcorn, defrosted
2 tbs (30g/1oz)	oyster sauce
2 tbsp	light soy sauce
6	spring onions, sliced diagonally into 2cm (1in) pieces
225g (8oz)	thread egg noodles, cooked according to instructions on the pack

1) Heat the oil in a wok or large pan. Stir-fry the onion and ginger for 2–3 minutes.
2) Add the prawns and five-spice powder and cook for a few minutes over a medium heat.
3) Stir in the beansprouts, sweetcorn, oyster sauce, soy sauce and spring onions and cook for a further few minutes.
4) Mix in the noodles, adjust the seasoning and heat through.

Healthy Eating Notes

Prawns and shellfish contain cholesterol, but the cholesterol found in food does not have a significant effect on your blood cholesterol level. This is because blood cholesterol is more influenced by the amount of saturated fat in the diet and other factors, such as being overweight.

Tandoori Prawns

Tandoori dishes are familiar favourites in Indian restaurants where the food is cooked quickly in a very hot clay oven. In this recipe, the prawns are cooked over a high heat in tandoori spices, which are available in the herbs section in supermarkets.

The prawns are served in warmed wholemeal pitta bread filled with shredded lettuce. There's no need to add butter or spread because the tandoori sauce is quite moist. You may like to accompany this with more salad and some Cucumber and Mint Raita (*see page 124*).

Preparation and cooking time: 15 minutes
Serves 2
Freezing: not recommended

2 tsp	tandoori spice mix
150g/5oz pot	low-fat natural yogurt
1 tsp	lemon juice
225g (8oz)	fresh or frozen prawns, defrosted if necessary
1 tsp	corn oil
1	small onion, finely chopped
2 tbs	chopped fresh coriander
2	wholemeal pitta breads, warmed
	a few lettuce leaves, shredded
1	fresh lemon, sliced

1) Blend together the spice mix, yogurt, lemon juice and prawns.
2) Heat the oil in a non-stick frying pan. Fry the onion over a medium heat until light brown.
3) Increase the heat to high and add the prawn mixture. Cook quickly, stirring frequently for about 5 minutes until the liquid is absorbed.
4) Stir in the coriander and remove from heat.
5) Slit the pitta breads open and stuff them with the lettuce. Add the tandoori prawns and serve with lemon slices.

Healthy Eating Notes

Choose wholemeal bread and wholemeal pitta bread to provide more fibre. Using low-fat natural yogurt in cooking helps to keep the overall fat content down.

15-Minute Mackerel

Fresh orange juice helps to counteract the richness of this oily fish. Delicious with a large chunk of crusty bread and mixed salad, or boiled new potatoes in their skins and steamed mixed vegetables.

Preparation and cooking time: 15 minutes
Serves 2
Freezing: not recommended

4   mackerel fillets (total weight around
     395g/14oz)
     juice of 2 fresh oranges
1   clove garlic, crushed
     salt and pepper

1) Preheat the grill to medium. Line the grillpan with foil and place each fillet skin side down on the foil.
2) Pour the orange juice over the mackerel and season with the garlic, salt and pepper.
3) Grill for 8–10 minutes, turning once after about 5 minutes.

Healthy Eating Notes
Although mackerel is high in fat, it is still a good source of omega-3 fatty acids. Try to eat oily fish once a week.

Oatmeal Herrings

This recipe reminds me of my home town, Edinburgh. It is often served as part of a hearty Scottish breakfast. Accompany this rich fish with mashed or boiled potatoes and peas or broccoli.

Preparation and cooking time: 20 minutes
Serves 4
Freezing: suitable

100g (4oz)	oats
	salt and pepper
4	herrings, filleted
1 tsp	corn oil
2	fresh lemons, sliced

1) Mix the oats with a little salt and pepper. Coat both sides of each herring with the oats, pressing firmly onto the fish.
2) Heat the oil in a non-stick frying pan. Place the fish, two at a time, skin side upwards, into the pan. Fry over a high heat until the underside is lightly brown.
3) Turn the fish over and cook the other side. Remove from the pan.
4) Cook the other two fish in the same way.
5) Blot the fish on kitchen paper and serve with fresh lemon.

Healthy Eating Notes
The traditional way to cook herrings in Scotland is to fry them. Make sure you pat them with kitchen towel to remove the excess oil.

Vegetarian Dishes

If you're about to flick past this chapter because you're not veg-etarian, then STOP! These recipes will introduce you to a wide variety of pulses and pastas as well as unusual ways of serving up vegetables. You can make a main meal of these nutritious dishes or simply team them up with meat or fish. And there's no need to soak dried pulses or do lots of chopping up and prepara-tion. Serve up Caribbean Rice or Pasta Shells with Olives and Oregano in less than 30 minutes.

Vegetarian dishes can be healthier, but this isn't always so, because dishes based on eggs and cheese can be high in fat. This chapter will show you how to choose reduced-fat versions of standard ingredients with no compromise on taste.

Recipes in this book have been specifically designed to cater for people who have diabetes or who wish to eat more healthily. If you are vegetarian, pulse vegetables such as beans and lentils provide a valuable source of protein. Together with starchy foods such as rice and pasta, you can prepare perfectly balanced meals. Pasta is particularly beneficial in diabetes because it has a more gradual effect on your blood glucose levels than many other carbohydrates.

A diet that contains plenty of fruit and vegetables is associat-ed with a reduced risk of heart disease and cancer. Beans and pulses are an excellent source of soluble fibre which has been shown to lower blood cholesterol. What's more, vegetables con-tain the antioxidant vitamins betacarotene and vitamin C, which are also protective against heart disease. All in all, vegetables are foods we should be eating more of. Use the recipes in this section to help you select the recommended amount of two large helpings of vegetables each day.

Pasta Shells with Olives and Oregano

A large portion lasts for days when your eyes are bigger than your stomach! This Italian meal needs only a side salad and bread to make it complete.

Preparation and cooking time: 20 minutes
Serves 3
Freezing: not recommended

255g (8oz)	pasta shells
1 tbs	olive oil
2	cloves garlic, crushed
1	onion, finely chopped
1	green pepper, diced
1½ tsp	dried oregano
55g (2oz)	pitted black olives
	salt and coarsely ground black pepper

1) Cook the pasta in lightly salted water according to the instructions on the packet.
2) Meanwhile, heat the oil in a large non-stick pan. Add the garlic, onion and green pepper and fry until the onions are light brown and the peppers are just cooked (about 5–7 minutes).
3) Stir in the oregano, olives, pasta and seasoning, and serve.

Healthy Eating Notes
Raw vegetables contain more vitamin C than cooked. Try to cook vegetables quickly so you retain as much of the vitamins as possible.

Macaroni and Cauliflower Cheese

Frozen cauliflower florets and an instant sauce sachet help to make this into a substantial, quick and easy meal. Choose a sauce mix to which you add milk, not water. This way you can use skimmed milk to help keep the fat down. If you can only find a sauce which is made up with boiling water, then bear in mind that the fat content may be a little higher. This is because the sauce mix may have been made with full-fat milk or added fat. Serve with vegetables such as broccoli, spinach or peas.

Preparation and cooking time: 35 minutes
Serves 4
Freezing: suitable

225g (8oz)	macaroni
395g (14oz)	frozen cauliflower florets
20g (¾oz) packet	instant white sauce mix
275ml (½ pint)	skimmed milk
115g (4oz)	half-fat Cheddar cheese, grated
	salt and pepper
½ tsp	French mustard
2	tomatoes, sliced (optional)

1) Cook the macaroni according to the instructions on the packet.
2) Meanwhile, steam or boil the cauliflower until just cooked.
3) Follow the instructions for making up the sauce, using the skimmed milk if required.
4) Stir in most of the cheese and season the sauce with the salt, pepper and mustard.
5) Preheat the grill to medium.
6) Mix the cooked, drained macaroni into the sauce and adjust the seasoning if necessary.
7) Put the mixture into a lightly greased flameproof dish. Sprinkle the remaining cheese and the sliced tomatoes on top. Grill until the cheese is brown and bubbling.

Healthy Eating Notes

Using skimmed milk and half-fat cheese makes this dish lower in fat than traditional recipes. If you don't like the taste of half- or reduced-fat cheeses, use a small amount of stronger-flavoured full-fat cheese. Low-fat alternatives can help you to reduce your fat intake as long as you don't eat more of them than your usual brand.

Vegetable Pasta in Tomato Sauce

I usually use pasta spirals or *penne* for this recipe. The pasta is not coated in a thick tomato sauce, but has just the right amount of tomato flavour and a hint of garlic. This is a dish you can serve on its own, especially since pasta is so filling. If anything, a side salad is all you need.

Preparation and cooking time: 30 minutes
Serves 4
Freezing: not recommended

285g (10oz)	pasta
1 tbsp	olive or rapeseed oil
1	clove garlic, crushed
255g (9oz)	canned chopped tomatoes
	pinch thyme
	pinch oregano
455g (1lb)	frozen mixed vegetables
	salt and pepper

1) Cook the pasta in lightly salted boiling water according to the instructions on the packet.
2) Meanwhile, heat the oil in a non-stick pan. Add the garlic and stir for a few seconds.
3) Pour in the tomatoes. Stir-fry until the tomatoes become soft and mushy (about 4–5 minutes).
4) Add the thyme, oregano, vegetables and seasoning. Cover and cook over a medium heat for about 5 minutes until the vegetables are cooked. Add a little hot water if the mixture begins to stick to the pan.
5) Mix in the drained, cooked pasta. Heat through and serve.

Healthy Eating Notes
Add a can of pulses like kidney beans or haricot beans to make this recipe a more substantial vegetarian meal.

Courgette and Mushroom Pizza

A crisp salad, ideally one with beans or sweetcorn, would make this into a delicious nutritious meal.

Preparation time: 10 minutes
Cooking time: 10 minutes
Serves 3
Freezing: suitable before cooking

1	ready-made pizza base, roughly 25cm (10in) diameter
2 tbsp	tomato purée
½ tsp	dried oregano
1	courgette, cut diagonally into thin slices
170g (6oz)	mushrooms, sliced
½	red pepper, cut into strips
	salt and pepper
85g (3oz)	reduced-fat Cheddar cheese, grated
1	tomato, sliced

1) Preheat the oven to 220°C/425°F/gas mark 7.
2) Brush the pizza bases with a little oil. Spread the tomato purée over the pizza base. Sprinkle the oregano on top.
3) Arrange the courgette slices, mushrooms and pepper strips over the pizza. Season with salt and pepper.
4) Add the cheese and decorate with the sliced tomato.
5) Place the pizza directly onto the oven shelf and cook for 15 minutes until the cheese is brown and bubbling.

Healthy Eating Notes
People with diabetes are encouraged to eat more starchy foods. Pizza is high in starchy carbohydrate. However, pizzas bought from fast-food outlets tend to be very high in fat as a lot of oil is used to make the base crisp and it is then smothered with full-fat mozzarella cheese. That's fine on occasions, but if you're a pizza-holic, then maybe experiment with this recipe. As an alternative, use different vegetable-based toppings such as sweetcorn and aubergines.

Speedy Pizza Baguettes

Even the kids can get stuck in to this fun and easy recipe. A bread base makes a nice change from traditional pizza bases. Try this with some sweetcorn and a mixed salad.

Preparation time: 10 minutes
Cooking time: 5 minutes
Serves 4
Freezing: not recommended

35cm (14in)	French baton loaf, cut into two and split lengthways
	a little olive oil, for brushing
2 tbs	tomato purée
½–1 tsp	oregano, as desired
60g (2oz)	reduced-fat Cheddar cheese, grated
2	tomatoes, sliced
8	pitted olives, halved

1) Preheat the grill to medium.
2) Brush each piece of the cut side of the bread with olive oil.
3) Spread the tomato purée evenly over the bread. Sprinkle the oregano on top.
4) Cover this with a layer of cheese. Arrange the tomato slices and olives over the cheese.
5) Grill on a wire rack for about 3–5 minutes until the cheese has melted, and serve immediately.

Healthy Eating Notes
You can combine foods so that if you eat a dish which is lower in fibre, you can add salad or vegetables. This recipe uses white bread. Although wholemeal and granary varieties of bread are preferable because they are higher in fibre, and hence good for a healthy digestive system, you don't need to choose them all the time.

Mexican Butter Beans with Rice

An unusual dish made from rice and vegetables – a perfect vegetarian meal with no need for any accompaniments.

Preparation and cooking time: 20 minutes
Serves 2
Freezing: suitable

115g (4oz)	long-grain rice, freshly cooked
140g (5oz)	canned butter beans, drained
2 tsp	oil
1	onion, finely chopped
1	clove garlic, crushed (optional)
1	green pepper, diced
1 tsp	red chilli powder, or to taste
115g (4oz)	chopped tinned tomatoes
85g (3oz)	low-fat soft cheese
2 tbs	chopped fresh coriander

1) Preheat the grill to medium.
2) Lightly grease a flameproof dish and place the cooked rice into this dish.
3) Put the beans on top of the rice.
4) Heat the oil and fry the onion, garlic (if used) and pepper. Cook for a few minutes to soften them.
5) Add the chilli and tomatoes and cook till the mixture becomes mushy.
6) Stir in the soft cheese and cover the beans with this sauce. Add most of the coriander, saving a little for garnish.
7) Grill for about a minute, garnish and serve immediately.

Healthy Eating Notes

Beans and rice both contain protein and serving them together like this helps to provide a balanced meal. All beans and lentils are rich in protein and soluble fibre and are low in fat.

Cottage Cheese and Vegetable Flan

No need to make your own pastry – simply buy some ready-made from the supermarket. This pastry freezes well, so you could purchase it in advance. If you're not an expert at rolling pastry to fit exactly into a flan ring, don't worry. A simple tip is to roll it out a little larger than you think you'll need and gently place it in the middle of the ring without stretching it. I use lots of fresh parsley in the filling which adds colour and a delicious herby flavour. Serve the flan with a fresh salad, such as Tomato and Coriander Salad (*see page 121*), and crusty bread for a light lunch.

Preparation time: 20 minutes
Cooking time: 35 minutes
Serves 4
Freezing: suitable

170g (6oz)	wholemeal shortcrust pastry
2 tsp	corn oil
8cm (3in)	stick of leek, sliced into rings
3	eggs, beaten
120ml (¼ pint)	skimmed milk
85g (3oz)	low-fat cottage cheese
	salt and black pepper
3 tbs	parsley, chopped
115g (4oz)	canned sweetcorn
115g (4oz)	frozen peas, boiled

1) Preheat the oven to 200°C/400°F/gas mark 6. Roll out the pastry onto a floured board.

2) Place a flan ring onto a baking tray. Gently lift the pastry off the board and into the flan ring. Allow the pastry to 'relax' for a few minutes. Prick the pastry all over with a fork to prevent it from rising and then bake it 'blind' (without any filling) in the centre of the oven for 15 minutes.

3) Meanwhile, heat the oil in a non-stick frying pan. Stir-fry the leek over a medium heat for 2–3 minutes.

4) In a bowl, beat the eggs and milk together. Add the cottage cheese, seasoning and parsley.

5) When the flan case has been cooking for 15 minutes, remove it from the oven. Arrange the leeks, sweetcorn and peas in the pastry case.

6) Cover with the egg mixture. Return this to the oven and bake for 35–40 minutes until the filling is set. Serve hot or cold.

Healthy Eating Notes

Standard flans are usually made with lots of full-fat cheese and whole milk. The cottage cheese in this recipe is very low in fat, yet still adds a soft creamy texture. Using skimmed milk also helps to keep the fat content down. Pastry is high in fat, so single-crust pies and flans like this are a better choice than double-crust ones.

Greek Potatoes with Feta Cheese

This is a main meal vegetarian choice which only needs some fresh mixed salad as an accompaniment.

Preparation time: 20 minutes
Cooking time: 30 minutes
Serves 4
Freezing: not recommended

900g (2lb)	potatoes, peeled and sliced
1	green pepper, diced
2	courgettes (about 225g/8oz), sliced
85g (3oz)	feta cheese, cut into small cubes
	freshly milled black pepper
1 tbs	Greek yogurt
2 tbs	skimmed milk
1 tbs	olive oil

1) Preheat the oven to 375°F/190°C/gas mark 5. Lightly grease a large ovenproof dish.
2) Boil the potatoes in lightly salted water for 10 minutes.
3) Layer the potatoes, pepper, courgettes and cheese into the dish, sprinkling some pepper in between.
4) Mix the yogurt with the milk and pour over the vegetables.
5) Drizzle the oil over the top, cover the dish with foil and bake until the vegetables are cooked (about 30 minutes).

Healthy Eating Notes

Feta cheese has a salty flavour which enables you to use the minimum amount of salt when preparing the rest of the dish. It is important to cut down on salt because it is associated with high blood pressure.

Stuffed Peppers

The traditional recipe for stuffed peppers can take around 40 minutes in the oven as well as preparation time for the rice filling. This method takes a less conventional but easy short cut. The peppers cook in boiling water while you prepare the filling, so no time is wasted. The meal can be on the table in around half an hour. Use this recipe for leftovers too. Almost anything can be stuffed into the cooked peppers; they look appetizing and one pepper per person is sufficient for a light lunch or supper. Serve with a mixed salad or Red Cabbage Coleslaw (*see page 120*) and extra bread.

Preparation and cooking time: 35 minutes
Serves 4
Freezing: not recommended

4	red peppers
2 tsp	corn oil
1	onion, finely chopped
2	cloves garlic, crushed
115g (4oz)	frozen peas
115g (4oz)	frozen sweetcorn
1 tsp	dried mixed herbs
	salt and black pepper
2 tbs	fresh parsley, chopped
115g (4oz)	long-grain rice, boiled
30g (1oz)	reduced-fat Cheddar cheese

1) Cut a circle round the stem end of each pepper and remove the seeds. Put this circle back onto the peppers to form a lid. Place the peppers upright in a saucepan half-filled with boiling water. Bring back to the boil, cover and cook for 10 minutes.
2) Meanwhile, heat the oil in a non-stick pan. Add the onion and garlic and fry over a gentle heat to soften.
3) Add the peas, sweetcorn and seasoning to the pan with a few tablespoons of hot water. Cover with a tight-fitting lid and cook the vegetables over a high heat for a few minutes.
4) Add the parsley and rice to the vegetables and stir gently until well mixed.
5) Spoon the rice mixture into the peppers, sprinkle with grated cheese and cover with the 'lids'.

Healthy Eating Notes
Vegetable dishes combined with a starchy carbohydrate like rice or pasta are generally quick and easy to make and can be just as nourishing as meat-based meals.

Curried Egg on Toast

A light snack consisting of spiced scrambled egg.

Preparation and cooking time: 10 minutes
Serves 2
Freezing: not recommended

1 tsp	rapeseed oil
3	spring onions, sliced
2	eggs, beaten
1	green chilli, deseeded and finely chopped
2 tbs	skimmed milk
	pinch turmeric
	pinch curry powder
3 tbs	chopped coriander leaves
	salt and pepper
2 slices	bread (preferably wholegrain), toasted, to serve

1) Heat the oil in a non-stick frying pan. Add the onions and fry gently for 1 minute.
2) Mix the eggs with the chilli, milk, turmeric and curry powder.
3) Add the egg mix to the pan and stir gently till the egg is cooked.
4) Mix in the coriander and add the seasoning if necessary. Serve immediately on top of the toast.

Healthy Eating Notes

Eggs contain cholesterol, but the cholesterol in foods has very little effect on your blood cholesterol. This is because blood cholesterol is more influenced by the amount of saturated fat (such as full-fat dairy products and fatty meat) in your diet.

Spanish Omelette

This is a wonderful dish to make when you have odd bits of peppers and tomatoes in the fridge. It's also a good way of using up leftover boiled potatoes. Vary it by adding tuna or ham if you prefer a non-vegetarian option. Serve cold – the Spanish way – with lots of toasted wholemeal or granary bread and a side salad.

Preparation and cooking time: 15 minutes
Serves 3
Freezing: not recommended

3	eggs, beaten
1 tbs	skimmed milk
	salt and pepper
1	small onion, finely chopped
¼	green pepper, finely chopped
1	tomato, chopped
1	potato (about 150g/5oz), peeled, chopped and boiled

1) Preheat the grill to medium. Mix the eggs with the milk and seasoning.
2) Brush a non-stick frying pan with a little oil. Heat the pan and add the onion and peppers. Fry for a few minutes to soften them.
3) Add the tomato, potato and the egg mixture. Stir for a few seconds and then allow the egg to set over a low heat for a few minutes.
4) Place the pan under the grill for two minutes until set and golden. Serve immediately.

Healthy Eating Notes

Eggs are a good source of protein and iron. Adding vegetables makes this into a more substantial and nutritious dish. Use a good non-stick frying pan so you minimize the amount of oil needed in preparation.

Caribbean Rice

A one-pot dish that needs 10 minutes of your time and is then left to cook completely on its own. Add the chillies according to your taste. If you prefer dishes with a bit more spice, choose hot Jamaican chilli peppers or Jamaican jerk seasoning, which are available in West Indian grocery shops. Use this recipe to add a starchy accompaniment to your main dish, or serve it as a main meal with a fresh side salad, such as Tomato and Coriander Salad (*see page 121*).

Preparation time: 10 minutes
Cooking time: 20 minutes
Serves 4
Freezing: suitable

1 tbs	corn oil
1	onion, finely chopped
170g (6oz)	canned chopped tomatoes in tomato juice
2	fresh green chillies, chopped or 2 tsp chilli sauce
	salt and pepper
420g (15oz) can	pigeon peas or red kidney beans, drained
225g (8oz)	rice
500ml (18fl oz)	boiling water

1) Heat the oil in a large saucepan with a lid. Fry the onions until they are browned (about 5 minutes).
2) Add the tomato, chillies and seasoning. Cook for a few minutes.
3) Gently stir in the peas (or beans), rice and boiling water.
4) Bring back to the boil, lower the heat, cover and cook for about 20 minutes until all the water is absorbed.

Healthy Eating Notes

You do not need to use brown rice in this recipe since there is already extra fibre in the added vegetables.

Herb Mushrooms on Toast

Preparation and cooking time: 10 minutes
Serves 3
Freezing: not recommended

1 tbs	olive oil
1	clove garlic, crushed
225g (8oz)	mushrooms, sliced
2 tbs	fresh thyme or basil, finely chopped
2 tbs	fresh parsley, finely chopped
	salt and coarsely ground black pepper
3	slices granary bread, toasted
1 tsp	sesame seeds

1) Heat the oil in a non-stick frying pan or wok. Add the garlic and mushrooms and stir-fry for a few minutes till the mushrooms are almost cooked.
2) Mix in the herbs and seasoning and cook for a further minute to soften the herbs.
3) Arrange the mushrooms on top of the toast and sprinkle with sesame seeds.

Healthy Eating Notes
A crunchy, low-calorie, low-fat, snappy supper dish or light vegetarian snack.

Vegetable Rice

Delicious with some crisp salad dressed with fat-free vinaigrette.

Preparation time: 10 minutes
Cooking time: 20 minutes
Serves 4
Freezing: not recommended

1 tbs	corn oil
1	onion, finely chopped
2	vegetable stock cubes, made up to 500ml (17½fl oz) with boiling water
225g (8oz)	long-grain rice
455g (1lb)	frozen mixed vegetables
½ tsp	ground turmeric
	salt and pepper

1) Heat the oil in a large saucepan with a lid. Fry the onion until browned (about 5 minutes).
2) Add all the other ingredients.
3) Bring back to the boil, lower the heat, cover and cook for about 20 minutes until all the water is absorbed.

Healthy Eating Notes
Vegetables and starchy foods together can make well-balanced, low-calorie meals.

Side Dishes and Accompaniments

Made the main part of the meal, got some pasta or potatoes on the boil, but still need a little something else? These accompaniments are designed to enhance the flavour of your dishes and to give you ideas on how to dress up vegetables when you want a change from steamed or boiled varieties. Choose dishes such as Hot Roasted Vegetables or Tomato and Coriander Salad to add colour, variety and essential nutrients.

Vegetables provide vitamins such as betacarotene (which is converted by the body to vitamin A) and vitamin C. Serving raw vegetables in salads or with dips is a great way of making sure you're getting enough of these nutrients. These 'antioxidant' vitamins are thought to protect against heart disease. Try to get into the habit of including at least one helping of vegetables or salad at every meal.

Bought salad dressings can add fat and calories to an otherwise healthy dish. In this chapter, you'll find ideas for salad dressings based on low-fat natural yogurt and lemon juice. Alternatively, choose fat-free dressings from the supermarket.

Several of the recipes contain beans, sweetcorn or peas. These provide an important source of soluble fibre which helps to control your blood glucose level. Further, these vegetables are a cheap, low-fat source of protein.

Creamy Broad Beans

A scrumptious way to serve up an otherwise bland vegetable. This fibre-rich dish can complement an otherwise low-fibre main course.

Preparation and cooking time: 10 minutes
Serves 2
Freezing: not recommended

200g (7oz)	frozen broad beans
55g (2oz)	medium-fat soft cheese
¼ tsp	dried mixed herbs
	salt and coarsely ground black pepper

1) Cook the beans in lightly salted boiling water in a covered pan. This should take 4–5 minutes.
2) Meanwhile, mix the cheese with the seasonings.
3) Stir the flavoured cheese into the drained beans, adjust the seasoning and heat through.

Healthy Eating Notes
Try to eat two large helpings of vegetables per day. Vegetables are good sources of the antioxidant vitamins A and C. Antioxidants are thought to protect against heart disease.

Sesame Green Beans

Tired of plain boiled vegetables? Make an interesting change with this recipe which you can use with any vegetables of your choice.

Preparation and cooking time: 10 minutes
Serves 4
Freezing: not recommended

455g (1lb)   frozen French beans
1 tsp   olive oil
2 tbs   sesame seeds

1) Boil the beans quickly till just cooked.
2) Heat the oil. Add the sesame seeds and then the drained, cooked beans. Stir till the beans are well coated with the seeds.

Healthy Eating Notes
Cook vegetables lightly in a minimum of water over a high heat to help preserve the vitamin C. Serving them immediately after cooking also helps to maintain the vitamin C content.

Curried Sweetcorn

Although this is a side dish, I must confess to having half the recipe as a main meal, served with low-fat natural yogurt and lots of naan bread – can you resist it? A yummy meal or snack that's on the table in 10 minutes. This side dish has quite a strong flavour, so use it to spice up an otherwise bland meal. It can be served on toast, or with any main dish and fresh salad.

Preparation and cooking time: 10 minutes
Serves 4
Freezing: not recommended

2 tsp	corn oil
1 tsp	cumin seeds
1 tbs	tomato purée
2 tsp	curry powder
326g (11½oz) can	sweetcorn
2	spring onions, sliced
2 tbs	fresh coriander, chopped

1) Heat the oil in a non-stick pan. Add the cumin seeds and let them pop for only a few seconds.
2) Stir in the tomato purée and curry powder, and blend together well over a low heat.
3) Mix in the sweetcorn, spring onions and coriander. Add a few tablespoons of hot water if you prefer more sauce, and serve hot.

Healthy Eating Notes

Vegetables are high in soluble fibre which helps you to control blood glucose levels more easily. This type of fibre has also been shown to lower blood fats such as cholesterol. Try to eat two large helpings of vegetables per day.

Barbecue Baked Beans

Baked beans are an excellent convenience food. This recipe adds variety to standard baked beans in a matter of minutes. A delicious accompaniment to any meal, or serve on granary toast or in jacket potatoes.

Preparation and cooking time: 5 minutes
Serves 2
Freezing: not recommended

425g (15oz) can	baked beans in tomato sauce
1 tbs	Worcester sauce
1 tbs	vinegar
1 tbs	soy sauce
	coarsely ground black pepper
pinch	mustard powder (optional)

Simply add all the ingredients to the beans in a pan, heat and serve.

Healthy Eating Notes

Baked beans are made from haricot beans which are a pulse vegetable. Pulses are high in soluble fibre. This type of fibre is slowly absorbed by the body, so it helps to minimize 'highs' and 'lows' in blood glucose.

Peas with Shallots

Preparation time: 5 minutes
Cooking time: 5 minutes
Serves 4
Freezing: not recommended

1	vegetable stock cube, made up to 150ml (¼ pint) with boiling water
340g (12oz)	frozen peas
8	button onions or shallots, peeled and halved
	good pinch marjoram
	salt and pepper

1) Put all the ingredients into a pan with a tight-fitting lid.
2) Bring back to the boil. Cover and simmer till the peas are cooked and the onions are softened.

Healthy Eating Notes
Try to have two large helpings of vegetables daily, and choose peas, beans or lentils often.

Southern Fries

If you love your chips but always thought they were too naughty to indulge in, here's a lower-fat way of having chips with extra flavour. Serve this dish with any meal you would normally like to have chips with. Reduce the amount of spices if you're cooking for young children who may prefer plainer flavours.

Preparation time: 5 minutes
Cooking time: 15 minutes
Serves 2
Freezing: not recommended

200g (7oz)	5 per cent fat oven chips
1 tsp	Cajun seasoning
¼ tsp	dried mixed herbs
½ tsp	dill pepper (optional)
	pinch of salt

1) Preheat the grill to medium. Line the grillpan with cooking foil.
2) Place the frozen chips in one layer on the grillpan.
3) Mix all the seasonings together.
4) Coat the chips with the seasoning and cook under the grill for 10–12 minutes, turning once during cooking.

Healthy Eating Notes
Chips bought from fish and chip shops can contain as much as 13 per cent fat. French fries sold in fast-food outlets have around 15 per cent fat. Choose reduced fat oven chips instead.

Creamed Potatoes with Cabbage

A delicious vegetable accompaniment to meat. The crunchy cabbage contrasts beautifully with the creamy texture of the potatoes. Serve in place of ordinary potatoes or rice.

Preparation and cooking time: 15 minutes
Serves 4
Freezing: not recommended

126g (4½oz) packet	instant mashed potato mix
2 tbs (40g)	half-fat crème fraîche
	salt and pepper
455g (1lb)	white cabbage, shredded and boiled
1 tbs	chopped fresh chives

1) Make up the mashed potato with boiling water according to the instructions on the packet. Blend in the half-fat crème fraîche and season.
2) Add the cabbage and chives and mix well.

Healthy Eating Notes
Mixing vegetables like cabbage with starchy foods such as potatoes is a great way of getting the kids to eat vegetables!

Hot Roasted Vegetables

This recipe combines traditional root vegetables, such as carrots, parsnips and swedes, and gives them a more Mediterranean flavour.

Preparation time: 20 minutes
Cooking time: 15 minutes
Serves 4
Freezing: not recommended

455g (1lb)	carrots, cut into matchsticks
455g (1lb)	parsnips, cut into matchsticks
455g (1lb)	swedes or turnips, diced
2 tsp	olive oil
2 tbs	pine nuts
1	clove garlic, crushed
	pinch dried herbs
2 tbs	chopped parsley
	salt and pepper

1) Preheat the oven to 375°F/190°C/gas mark 5. Lightly grease an ovenproof dish.
2) Cook the vegetables for 3–4 minutes in boiling water.
3) Drain the vegetables and mix with the other ingredients.
4) Put the mixture into the dish and roast in the oven for about 15 minutes.

Healthy Eating Notes

People in the UK eat less fruit and vegetables than is recommended for good health. Try to eat five portions of fruit and vegetables (not counting potatoes) a day. Vegetables are low in calories, high in fibre and most are fat-free. Preparing dishes such as this makes a refreshing change from boiled vegetables.

Three Bean Salad

This fibre-rich side dish is a great accompaniment to a low-fibre meal. Serve it with quiches and pizzas, or simply with a jacket potato filled with cottage cheese.

Preparation time: 10 minutes
Serves 6
Freezing: not recommended

420g (15oz) can	chickpeas, drained
420g (15oz) can	kidney beans, drained
420g (15oz) can	blackeye beans, drained
3	spring onions, chopped
2 tbs	chopped parsley

FOR THE DRESSING

4 tbs	low-fat natural yogurt
2 tbs	cider vinegar
2 tbs	olive oil
	salt and pepper

1) Add the beans to the spring onions and parsley in a large salad bowl.
2) Put the dressing ingredients into a screw-top jar, cover with a tight-fitting lid and shake well.
3) Pour the dressing over the beans. Chill in the refrigerator and stir just before serving.

Healthy Eating Notes
The low-fat yogurt dressing adds flavour without the calories of traditional salad dressings.

Potato Wedges

Preparation time: 10 minutes
Cooking time: 15 minutes
Serves 4
Freezing: not recommended

3   baking potatoes, washed and scrubbed
2 tbs   rapeseed or olive oil
2 tsp   Chinese five-spice powder or dill pepper
    salt and freshly ground black pepper

1) Preheat the grill to high and line the grillpan with aluminium foil.
2) Cut each potato lengthways into 8 wedges. Boil in lightly salted water until just cooked. Drain.
3) Lightly grease the foil and put the cooked potatoes into the grillpan. Season with the five-spice powder and pepper.
4) Drizzle or brush the oil over the wedges and brown for 5–10 minutes under a hot grill. Serve immediately.

Healthy Eating Notes
Boiling, brushing with oil and grilling potatoes can still produce crisp, golden potato wedges which taste every bit as good as the traditional deep-fried version – without the extra fat!

Minted Carrot Salad

Preparation time: 10 minutes
Serves 4
Freezing: not recommended

4	carrots, diced
1 tsp	mint sauce
55g (2oz)	raisins

1) Simply mix and serve.

Healthy Eating Notes

Although dried fruits are high in sugar, it is perfectly acceptable
to use them if you have diabetes.

Red Cabbage Coleslaw

A filling portion size to complement any meal.

Preparation time: 15 minutes
Serves 4
Freezing: not recommended

225g (8oz)	red cabbage, shredded or grated
3	carrots, grated
3	spring onions, sliced
115ml (4oz)	reduced-calorie mayonnaise

1) Simply mix all the ingredients together and serve!

Healthy Eating Notes
The reduced-calorie mayonnaise helps to keep the fat lower than standard coleslaw. If you want to get it down further, choose a low-fat natural yogurt or fat-free vinaigrette instead.

Tomato and Coriander Salad

A refreshing accompaniment to any meal.

Preparation time: 10 minutes
Serves 4
Freezing: not recommended

455g (1lb)	tomatoes, thinly sliced
4	spring onions, finely sliced
15g (½oz) packet	fresh coriander, chopped
	coarsely ground black pepper
	lemon juice, to taste

1) Simply mix all the ingredients together and serve.

Healthy Eating Notes

Tomatoes are rich in betacarotene which is converted into vitamin A in the body. Vegetables, especially raw vegetables, are also good sources of vitamin C. Vitamins A, C and E are antioxidant vitamins which are thought to help in the prevention of heart disease.

Five-Minute Potato Salad

Preparation time: 5 minutes
Serves 4
Freezing: not recommended

540g (19oz) can	unpeeled potatoes, drained
140ml (5fl oz)	low-fat natural yogurt
3 tbs	fresh chives, snipped
	salt and coarse black pepper

1) Cut the potatoes into halves.
2) Mix the yogurt with the chives and seasoning.
3) Dress the potatoes with the yogurt mixture and serve chilled.

Healthy Eating Notes
Unpeeled potatoes help to provide fibre, and low-fat yogurt makes an excellent substitute for full-fat, or even reduced-calorie, mayonnaise.

Salsa Sauce

Add a touch of Mexico to your meals with this crunchy, lightly spiced sauce. Serve hot or cold as a relish for hamburgers or lean grilled chops.

Preparation and cooking time: 15 minutes
Serves 4
Freezing: suitable

1 tsp	corn oil
1	clove garlic, crushed
1	small onion, finely chopped
½	green pepper, diced
200g (7oz)	canned chopped tomatoes in tomato juice
¼ tsp	red chilli powder

1) Heat the oil in a non-stick frying pan.
2) Add the garlic, onion and pepper, and fry gently for about 4–5 minutes.
3) Add the tomatoes and chilli. Lower the heat and simmer for about 5 minutes, stirring occasionally.

Cucumber and Mint Raita

Preparation time: 10 minutes
Serves 4
Freezing: not recommended

500g (17½oz)	carton low-fat natural yogurt
1 tbs	chopped fresh mint
½ tsp	coarsely ground black pepper
½	cucumber, grated

1) Season the yogurt with the mint and pepper. Chill.
2) Just before serving, stir in the cucumber.

Healthy Eating Notes
Choose low-fat dairy products (such as low-fat yogurt, low-fat fromage frais, reduced-calorie mayonnaise) wherever possible. Low-fat dairy foods can help you to cut down on your saturated fat intake so long as you don't eat more of them than the full-fat version.

Instant Mint Chutney

A runny chutney which is great when used as a dipping sauce for chicken drumsticks or sausages (lower-fat ones, of course!). If you prefer a thicker chutney, simply add less water.

Preparation time: 5 minutes
Serves 3
Freezing: not recommended

2 tbsp	tomato ketchup
1 tsp	mint sauce
¼–½ tsp	red chilli powder
2 tbsp	cold water

1) Simply mix all the ingredients together!

Crunchy Cucumber Relish

Preparation time: 10 minutes
Serves 4
Freezing: not recommended

1   cucumber, diced
40g (1½oz)   chopped nuts, e.g. peanuts
1 tbs   lemon juice
salt and coarsely ground black pepper

1) Simply mix and serve.

Healthy Eating Notes
Nuts and seeds are a good source of vitamins and minerals, especially vitamin E and zinc. These are needed in small amounts for good health.

Desserts

Banana and Chocolate Pie and Pears in Blackcurrant Sauce are only a couple of the tempting treats you'll find in this chapter. Having diabetes doesn't mean saying goodbye to those sweet endings to your meals. All sorts of desserts can be incorporated into a healthy diet, particularly if you choose appropriate ingredients. Half-fat creams, low-fat instant dessert mixes and fresh fruit have been suggested in these recipes as they help to reduce the fat and sugar content of traditional puds. To cut down even further on fat, try using virtually fat-free fromage frais or low-fat natural yogurt.

Base desserts on fresh fruit as often as possible and try to eat three pieces of fruit every day.

Speedy Trifle

One of those desserts that can be made in advance and is a kids' favourite, this recipe makes use of an instant custard mix so there's no need to worry about disguising those lumps. You can choose any fruit, but remember to buy the fruit canned in natural juice or fruit juice, rather than in syrup. If you have more time, you may want to make a sugar-free jelly and pour this over the fruit. Allow it to set in the refrigerator for about 45 minutes, then add the custard and cream.

Preparation time: 25 minutes
Serves 6
Freezing: not recommended

415g (14½oz) can	fruit cocktail in natural juice
8	trifle sponge fingers or 4 trifle sponges (approx. 100g/4oz)
70g (2½oz) packet	low-fat instant custard mix
140ml (5fl oz)	half-fat whipping cream
2	kiwi fruits, sliced

1) Drain the fruit juice from the fruit cocktail and set aside.
2) Arrange the drained fruit and sponge cake in the bottom of a large pudding bowl.
3) Pour the reserved fruit juice over the sponge cake. Place the bowl in the refrigerator to chill.
4) Meanwhile, make up the custard with boiling water as indicated on the packet. Allow to cool.
5) Pour the custard over the sponge and fruit mixture, and put the bowl back into the refrigerator.
6) Whip the cream and spread it over the chilled custard.
7) Decorate with the kiwi fruit and serve chilled.

Healthy Eating Notes

Standard trifle ingredients have been replaced with lower-fat and reduced-sugar versions by incorporating low-fat custard, canned fruit in natural juice and half-fat cream.

Banana and Chocolate Pie

No rolling of pastry, no baking. All you need is a knife and a whisk and you can create this scrumptious dessert in 15 minutes.

This recipe is far lower in fat than standard creamy pies, but to keep an eye on your fat intake, serve it after a low-fat main course, such as Vegetable Pasta in Tomato Sauce (*see pages 82–3*), which has less than 5 per cent fat.

Preparation time: 15 minutes
Serves 8
Freezing: suitable

49g (1¾oz) packet	sugar-free chocolate-flavour whipped dessert mix, e.g. Angel Delight
275ml (½ pint)	skimmed milk
3	bananas, sliced or mashed
18cm (7in)	bought pastry case
90ml (3fl oz)	half-fat whipping cream
½	bar chocolate flake, crumbled
20g (¾oz)	chopped nuts

1) Make up the whipped dessert with the skimmed milk according to the instructions on the packet.
2) Put the bananas into the pastry case. Cover with the made-up dessert.
3) Whip the cream and layer on top.
4) Sprinkle the chocolate crumbs and nuts over the cream. Chill and serve.

Healthy Eating Notes

Although the bought pastry case is just as high in fat and sugar as ordinary sweet pastry, this recipe uses sugar-free mousse for the filling and half-fat cream for the topping. This makes it lower in fat than standard creamy pies.

Hot Bananas with Almonds

A naturally sweet, easy dessert that takes just over five minutes to prepare. The bananas are split, flavoured with almonds and raisins and then sandwiched together. They are cooked in their own skin, so all the juices are preserved. This is a great way to prepare bananas if you are planning a barbecue, as they can be cooked on the charcoal in their skins. Since each banana is served wrapped in its parcel of foil, it's also a fun and sneaky way to get kids to eat fruit!

Preparation time: 5–10 minutes
Cooking time: 20 minutes
Serves 4
Freezing: not recommended

4	bananas
2 tbs	lemon juice
30g (1oz)	flaked almonds
30g (1oz)	raisins

1) Preheat the oven to 220°C/425°F/gas mark 7.
2) Make one lengthways slit in each banana, keeping the skin as intact as possible. Sprinkle on the lemon juice.
3) Stuff the almonds and raisins into each banana.
4) Cover the whole banana with foil.
5) Repeat this with all the bananas. Place them directly onto the rack in the oven. Cook for 20–25 minutes till they are soft.

Healthy Eating Notes
People in the UK eat far less fruit than is recommended for health. Try to eat three pieces of fruit per day. Fruit is high in the antioxidant vitamins (A and C), which have been shown to be protective against heart disease.

Pineapple Muesli Crumble

No chopping of fruit, no tedious preparation of crumble toppings. Ready-made ingredients help you to prepare this hot pud
in a jiffy. You can use a variety of accompaniments, depending on
the occasion. Low-fat yogurt, low-fat custard made up from a
sachet and ice-cream are much lower in fat than fresh cream.
You could also try a spoonful of fromage frais or Greek yogurt.
The fruit in this recipe provides ample sweetness for the dish, so
there is no need to use muesli with added sugar, whether or not
you have diabetes.

Preparation time: 10 minutes
Cooking time: 25 minutes
Serves 6
Freezing: suitable

2	large bananas, sliced
425g (15oz) can	crushed pineapple in pineapple juice
140g (5oz)	sugar-free muesli
1 tbsp	corn oil

1) Preheat the oven to 180°C/350°F/gas mark 4. Lightly grease an ovenproof dish.
2) Put the bananas, pineapple and juice into the bottom of the dish.
3) Mix the muesli with the oil. Pour this mixture over the fruit.
4) Cover with foil and bake in the centre of the oven for 20 minutes. Remove the foil and cook for a further 5 minutes.

Healthy Eating Notes
Muesli contains dried fruit, oats and nuts. Oats are particularly beneficial in diabetes because they contain soluble fibre which helps to slow down the rise in blood glucose after meals.

Baked Apple

Preparation time: 10 minutes
Cooking time: 30–40 minutes
Serves 2
Freezing: not recommended

2	cooking apples, cored
30g (1oz)	raisins
¼ tsp	mixed spice
¼ tsp	ground cinnamon

1) Preheat the oven to 180°C/350°F/gas mark 4. Lightly grease an ovenproof dish.
2) Make a cut in the skin around the middle of each apple. Place the apples in the dish.
3) Mix the raisins with the spices and fill each apple with this mixture.
4) Cover the dish with foil and bake in the centre of the oven till cooked (about 30–40 minutes).

Healthy Eating Notes
The raisins are sweet enough to flavour this recipe without needing to add sugar. Dried fruits are also a good source of iron.

Biscuit and Strawberry Pudding

This dessert is high in fat, so save it for special occasions.

Preparation time: 20 minutes
Serves 6
Freezing: not recommended

140g (5oz)	semi-sweet biscuits (e.g. Marie, Rich Tea), crushed
284ml (10fl oz) carton	half-fat whipping cream, whipped
395g (14oz)	strawberries, sliced

1) Put half the biscuits into the bottom of a large, shallow dessert dish, or into six individual glass serving dishes.
2) Cover this with a thin layer of cream.
3) Arrange half the strawberries on top of the cream.
4) Repeat steps 1–3. Chill and serve.

Healthy Eating Notes
Try to base dessert dishes on fresh fruit. Cut down on fat and calories by choosing half-fat cream, virtually fat-free fromage frais or low-fat natural yogurt.

Pears in Blackcurrant Sauce

Fruit-based puddings are generally healthier choices for every-one. Here's a delicious speedy alternative to the usual pears in red wine. To save time, you can use canned pear halves in natural juice and omit step 1.

Preparation and cooking time: 15 minutes
Serves 4
Freezing: not recommended

2	firm dessert pears, peeled, halved and cored
1 piece	stem ginger, quartered (optional)
	few drops lemon juice
½ tsp	cornflour
2 tbs (about 30g/1oz)	reduced-sugar blackcurrant jam

1) Put the pears, ginger (if used) and lemon juice into a pan with 150ml (5fl oz) of boiling water. Bring back to the boil, cover and simmer for about 10 minutes until the pears are cooked.

2) Meanwhile, mix the cornflour into a paste with a little cold water. Heat the jam gently with 60ml (2fl oz) of water and the cornflour paste. Bring this slowly to the boil, whilst stirring, and allow to thicken. Remove from the heat.

3) Arrange the pears, curved side up, on a serving dish. Pour the sauce over the pears and serve chilled.

Healthy Eating Notes

Look out for reduced-sugar jam and canned pears in natural juice to cut down on sweetness and sugar.

Apricot Rice Pudding

Traditional baked rice puds can take an hour or more to cook in the oven. Make use of this short-cut recipe which uses a can of ready-made low-fat rice pudding.

Preparation and cooking time: 15 minutes
Serves 4
Freezing: not recommended

30g (1oz)	ready-to-eat dried apricots, chopped
1	apple, peeled, cored and chopped
1	cinnamon stick
	pinch of nutmeg
425g (15oz) can	low-fat rice pudding

1) Place the apricots, apple, cinnamon and nutmeg in a pan with 150ml (5fl oz) boiling water. Bring back to the boil, cover and simmer till the apple is soft (about 5 minutes).
2) Add the rice pudding and mix well. Serve hot or chilled.

Healthy Eating Notes
If you have a poor appetite, a milk pudding can be a nourishing addition to your meals.

Index

alcohol xiii–xiv
almonds, hot bananas with 132–3
apple, baked 136
apple and cucumber, prawns with 11
apple, pork with spiced 46–7
apricot rice pudding 140

baked apple 136
baked beans, barbecue 110
baked tomato and olive salad 17
banana and chocolate pie 130–31
bananas, hot with almonds 132–3
barbecue baked beans 110
beef:
    curry 38–9
    stew 36–7
biscuit and strawberry pudding 137
blackcurrant sauce, pears in 138–9
blackened fish 60–61
blood pressure, high viii
blood sugar (glucose) v, vii, viii, ix, x
bread, garlic 14
British Diabetic Association xvi
broad bean salad, ham and 21
broad beans, creamy 106
burgers, spicy lamb 40–41
butter beans, Mexican with rice 88–9

cabbage, creamed potatoes with 113
Caribbean rice 100–101

carrot salad, minted 119
carrot soup, lentil and 8
cashew nuts, chicken with 22–3
cauliflower cheese 80–81
chicken:
    lemony roast 28–9
    liver and fennel 30–31
    wings, chilli 4–5
    with cashew nuts 22–3
    pulau 24–5
chilli:
    chicken wings 4–5
    con carne 44–5
chocolate pie, banana and 130–31
chow mein, prawn 70–71
chutney, instant mint 125
cocktail:
    florida 16
    kebabs with yogurt dip 6–7
    tuna 9
cod in parsley sauce 54–5
coleslaw, red cabbage 120
coriander salad, tomato and 121
cottage cheese flan 90–91
cottage pie 42–3
courgette and mushroom pizza 84–5
cream:
and mustard sauce, salmon in 64–5
    tagliatelle with ham and 50–51
creamed potatoes with cabbage 113